TANTRIC
QUEST

TANTRIC QUEST

An Encounter with Absolute Love

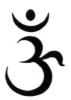

Daniel Odier

Translated from the French by Jody Gladding

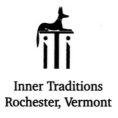

Inner Traditions
Rochester, Vermont

Inner Traditions International
One Park Street
Rochester, Vermont 05767
www.InnerTraditions.com

First English edition published in the United States in 1997

Originally published in French under the title *Tantra: L'initiation d'un occidental à l'amour absolu.*

Library of Congress Cataloging-in-Publication Data

Odier, Daniel, 1945–
  [Tantra. English]
  Tantric quest : an encounter with absolute love / Daniel Odier;
  translated from the French by Jody Gladding.
      p.   cm.
  ISBN 0-89281-620-1 (alk. paper)
  1. Spiritual life—Tantrism. I. Title.
BL1283.85204513 1997
294.5'514—dc21   97-1786
                                            CIP

Printed and bound in Canada

10 9 8 7 6 5 4 3 2

Type design and layout by Peri Champine
This book was typeset in Bitstream Charter with Delphian as the display typeface.

For Kalou Rinpoche and Devi,
my masters

In truth, every body is the universe.

Mahanirvana tantra

INTRODUCTION

Shivaic Tantrism of Kashmir occupies an extraordinary place in the history of thought. Originating seven thousand years ago in the Indus valley, this mystical, scientific, and artistic movement of the Dravidian culture encompasses all human potential and assigns a special place to the adept who is totally engaged in the way of knowledge. Tantrism is probably the only ancient philosophy that has survived all historical upheavals, invasions, and influences to reach us intact by uninterrupted transmission from master to disciple, and the only one, as well, to retain the image of the Great Goddess without inverting the power between woman and man to favor the latter. Entire lineages have followed great women masters, and still today, numerous yoginis transmit this age-old wisdom. Great male masters have often retained the custom of initiating a female disciple as a way to draw from the very source of power.

The Dravidians, seafaring people, built the great cities of Mohenjo Daro and Harappa. Their civilization extended from the Indus valley, in what is now Pakistan, to the Red Sea and the Mediterranean. The invasion of Aryan tribes from the Ukraine, three thousand years ago, put an end to the Dravidian civilization, but the formidable mystical movement underlying it survived. The masters fled the occupied citadels and took up residence in the countryside and in inaccessible places throughout the Himalayan mountain chain.

Shivaic Tantrism reemerged openly at the beginning of the fourth century A.D. in Kashmir, located, naturally, at the crossroads of the great cultural and commercial routes. Kashmir was part of the mysterious country of Oddiyana, situated between Afghanistan, India, and Pakistan. It included the valley of Swât, birthplace of numerous Mahasiddhas and dakinis, great Tantric initiators who spread the doctrine throughout the rest of India, Nepal, China, and Tibet.

Shiva and Shakti, the inseparable divine couple, are the gods of the ecstatic dance and the creators of the yoga that allows adepts to rediscover the divine at the root of their own minds by opening the heart. In the West, we usually move about in a universe based on duality: In the beginning, "God separated the light from the darkness" (Genesis 1:3). It is essential to understand that Tantrism stands apart from all separation between light and darkness, humans and gods. It is non-dualistic. It considers the mind to be fundamentally illuminated. Thus, the mind harbors all divinity. It is the source from which all is born and to which all returns: all phenomena, all differentiations, all mythical and divine creations, all sacred texts, all teachings, all illusory dualities.

The work of tantrikas, Tantric adepts, is thus to dispense with the illusory obscurities from which the ego, which originated these distinctions in the first place, arises. They then realize the nature of their own intrinsically pure minds. In dualistic thought, we imagine God outside of ourselves and direct our desire for union toward the exterior. In nonduality, the quest is reversed. Mystic energy is directed toward the interior, toward the mind. To realize the nature of the mind is thus the highest accomplishment. From this perspective, the passions are no longer considered antagonistic to mystical life. Their energy is used directly by the tantrika, and it is in this great conflagration that ardor dissolves the ego.

Needless to say, the widespread image that reduces Tantrism to vague sexual techniques meant to miraculously liberate their practitioners, under the guise of spirituality, has nothing to do with Shivaism. Such practices—ineffectual, since they are not based on true yoga asceticism, which depends upon the triple mastery of the breath, mental emptiness, and bodily processes—are, at best, only harmless deviances, not so harmless if manipulation is involved.

Tantrism is a way of total love, which leads to the freedom to be. It is through this story of my encounter with a great yogini and her teachings that I invite you to share this marvelous experience.

I

Her dark skin perfumed and oiled, the yogini seemed to float in space, her legs pulled up into Vs on either side of her body, her expression illuminated. Her open sex, where all originates and returns, radiated golden light, which met the blue of the sky. I remained fascinated, seated silently next to the Chinese yogi who had welcomed me into his hermitage. The yogini, his companion, at the same time close and distant, body and spirit, power and gift, steady in her yoga posture, was the incarnation of the extraordinary potential of realization.

The yogi practiced both Tantrism and Ch'an, or Zen, of Chinese origin, following the example of the sixth-century Indian master, Bodhidharma, heir to the two lineages. The twenty-eighth patriarch after the historical Buddha, and the first Patriarch of Zen, Bodhidharma arrived in China by sea and established himself in the famous monastery at Shao-lin, where he spent nine years meditating in front of a rock wall before transmitting the *dharma* (the doctrine) to Hui-k'o, the Second Chinese Patriarch. The dialogue between Bodhidharma and the Chinese emperor Wu of the Liang dynasty, a defender of Buddhism who was left puzzled by the laconic responses of the First Patriarch, is still well known:

"What merit have I gained by supporting Buddhism and building so many temples?"

"None."

"What is the highest meaning of the Sacred Truth?"

"Nothing is sacred. All is void."

"Who is this who is facing me?"

"I don't know."

The doctrine of Bodhidharma has four tenets:

  direct transmission, over and above the Buddhist
    scriptures,
  a foundation not in the texts but in the experience of
    Awakening,
  revelation to each individual disciple of the nature of
    his or her mind,
  contemplation of one's true nature, which is the
    Buddha nature.

We can see that these four main points correspond to the teachings of Tantric Shivaism, which are their source.

At the time of my departure, my host gave me a copy of his commentary and translation of the Vijnanabhairava Tantra, one of the most ancient and profound of the Tantric texts, held in high esteem by the Shivaites. This Tantra gave me my first glimpse of the goddess and the way that led me to meet my master, the Shivaic yogini Devi, seven years later, on the other side of India.

My interest in Buddhism, Hinduism, and Tantrism had declared itself very early. As a Protestant student in an austere abbey at the foot of a high rock wall, I had discovered and become fascinated with the splendors of religious services, where I sometimes served in a crimson vestment trimmed with lace. A resident bishop, a fabulous treasure given to the abbey by Charlemagne, a fantastically talented organist, and an excellent choir of which I was part captivated me from the start. Very strict studies and 6:30 mass every morning, followed by half an hour of work before breakfast did what was necessary to build character. Corporal punishment was still practiced—an assortment of various tortures like kneeling for an hour, arms crossed, a dictionary on each hand. Sometimes the periods of free time were replaced with interminable hours of copying out the texts of Latin authors or pages from the *Petit Larousse*. At night, the huge dormitories were crossed in silence; strange meetings took place on the roofs, where we went to smoke and talk about love. In such places there was terrible loneliness, a sometimes unbearable lack of affection, suicide attempts, forced vocations, bloody fights from which I still have scars, and sordid stories of love. Nevertheless, the excellence of the teachers; their devotion; the personality of the director, who charged around on his motorbike, cassock billowing in the wind; and the general atmosphere of the place had me seduced.

In that same period of my life, a friend of my parents, a beautiful and rebellious painter who looked a bit like Ava Gardner and drove a red Alfa Romeo, began to encourage my passion for art in general and painting in particular. On her advice, I applied myself to painting and drawing. I returned to Geneva, where I was born, to continue my studies at another religious college, a much less strict one, even though one of our teachers loved to pass "the dynamo" to us—a device that could explode powerfully, though it was supposedly harmless.

I was able to return home to my parents each weekend. I took those opportunities to visit my mentor and talk to her for hours about painting and music and literature. I was madly in love with her. For my sixteenth birthday, she took me out to dinner alone at a luxurious restaurant. Seated in big comfortable chairs, we dined by candlelight. I thought only of how I was going to declare my love for her. That evening, she gave me the *Bhagavad-Gita,* one of the key Hindu texts, with a commentary by Sri Aurobindo, a great sage profoundly influenced by Tantrism. This "spiritual" gift only fanned the flame, and my heart began to resemble one of the three lotuses printed on the saffron dust cover of this highly regarded collection, many titles of which I would go on to discover. As for my passion, it remained a secret. As consolation, I was later given access to *The Divine Life* in five volumes, the master work of this great Indian philosopher. Then, still secretly in love, I received the three volumes of *Essays on Zen Buddhism* by D. T. Suzuki. My only passion now was to become a mystic. The priests came to my aid. Twice they confiscated my works by Aurobindo, which I immediately repurchased. Without them, would I have clung to these difficult books with so much tenacity?

Some time later, my love urged me to enter my work in the competitive examination at the Roman Academy of

Fine Arts, and I won a scholarship. In Rome, I finally experienced love with a young actress, a member of the Carmelo Bene troupe. It was also there that I tasted total freedom in the marvelous ochres, the gardens, the fountains, the scent of pine and eucalyptus, and the heat of the crowd where artists from all countries passed each other. This was the life I'd dreamed about all those cold nights during the years of boarding school in the cramped atmosphere of a country I felt had closed in on itself.

Of course, I'd brought with me my favorite books, completely dog-eared, and tried in vain to reconcile a marvelous, frenetic life with the lessons of wisdom of the great Zen masters. I experienced a violent and destructive passion and then a more harmonious love. I left Rome to settle in Sperlonga, a small white village that rose above the sea, and, neglecting painting for a bit, I began to work on my first novel.

On leaving the Academy of Fine Arts of Rome, I met the art editor Albert Skira. Fascinated with Tibetan painting, I proposed a book to him. Skira, touched by my enthusiasm, which was equaled only by my ignorance, had me take some art photography classes, and, thus equipped with what I needed, I started on the route to India to photograph paintings. I had even decided to find a way of reconciling my fantastic appetite for life with the practice of wisdom, which reading alone had not done for me and which kept me in a state of constant imbalance. My impassioned sensual thirst could not achieve equilibrium with my spiritual aspirations. I was constantly torn by the spirit/flesh duality, and I didn't see how to arrive at this serenity that completely fascinated me, being so deeply rooted in the reality of life. I didn't seem to have the soul of an ascetic. I couldn't see myself living in a cave. I wanted everything; beauty, art, flesh, emotional intensity, love, sensuality, *and* spirituality. It seemed to me that our system of Western thought, based on separation, sacrifice, original sin, guilt, and suffering, could not answer my expectations, in spite of the glimmers of brilliance I had discovered among the pre-Socratic Greek philosophers and among certain Christian mystics.

In the autumn of 1968, I arrived in the green foothills of the Himalayas. I was twenty-three years old. I was looking for a master who could help me penetrate where texts and intellectual searching could no longer guide me. I was looking for a way that no longer divided aspirations and compartmentalized quests, a way to use the fabulous energy of passion reconciled, finally, with the divine.

I had naively allowed myself all of a year for intense practice, and I had decided to let the Shakti guide me to the one who would help me penetrate the heart of the Tantric doctrine. Little did I suspect that this itinerary would take twenty-five years of asking questions, of dreams, of practice, of failures and successes, anguish and joy, and then finally of abandonment, which, without warning, in 1993, would emerge into what I no longer imagined possible: initiation into Mahamudra and the opening of The Heart.

Mahamudra, or "Great Seal," is the last initiation of the Kargyupa school of Tibetan Buddhism, over the course of which the master presents to the disciple the nature of his true mind and transmits to him the power of immediate realization. If the operation succeeds, it is a non-way *(anupaya)* as opposed to all the gradual stages and preliminary initiations. Once the nature of the mind is realized, there is no longer any duality and thus no way to pursue, no end to attain, nothing more to do than to let things be by keeping the mind in its natural state—at peace, awakened, divine.

2

From those first weeks in the Himalayas, I sent off test film of my photographs of Tibetan art, which my editor found satisfactory. What remained, then, was to penetrate the mystery of this type of painting and to account for its profound meaning. For that, I would need to meet the masters.

A long pilgrimage had me traveling up and down a good part of the Himalayan chain, going from monastery to monastery to photograph the most beautiful paintings, sometimes walking for a week or two to reach isolated spots. Little by little, I penetrated the extremely rich and subtle symbolism of this magical cartography, which mapped the states of consciousness traversed during the course of different forms of meditation. It was now necessary to leave the field of theory for practice.

After six months of hard work, I decided to go back down to New Delhi to entrust the fruits of my labor to a diplomat, who would deliver it by hand to my editor. I would then have a good year for writing the text, and, with the photography for the book behind me, I planned to follow the teachings of some great Tibetan master. My initial work had given me opportunities to meet with the highest authorities of the various schools. Now I needed to go back to see those who had left the greatest impression and ask one of them to take me on as a disciple.

Just before my train entered the Delhi station, the power was interrupted and the lights went off for a few minutes. When they came back on, I realized that my suitcase of film and my camera had disappeared. In a state of shock, I filed a complaint with the station police and launched into a desperate search.

Furious and worn out, I spent the night hunting through all the nearby garbage cans, questioning in vain those who slept on the street, in the hope that the thief had abandoned my film bag. I thought about those long and difficult treks, about the marvels I had uncovered, and, occasionally, about the cost of enduring patience. Here were hundreds of kilometers I'd crossed by foot, countless meetings, and hard-won permissions, and above all a treasure of many thousands of negatives, vanishing forever. A band of shrewd, resourceful street urchins who knew their way around came to my aid, and I promised them a big reward. Dawn arrived, and not the least trace of the film had been found.

Bitter and disappointed at watching my big chance to publish a book with a great editor disappear, I decided to stay in Delhi for ten or fifteen days. The first thing I did was take a room with a bath in a luxury hotel in Janpath to taste a pleasure I hadn't known for months. I had bathed in rivers, sacred and otherwise, in streams and lakes, but not once in a bathtub. By this time, I was wearing several protective cords around my neck from all my meetings with lamas and rinpoches. I ran the bath very hot and, quivering with pleasure, slipped into the deep, claw-footed tub. Immersed so suddenly in the hot water, the cords began to shrink, and it was only by pulling on them with both hands that I escaped strangulation by too much protection. It was a rough landing, very Tibetan in substance, and signifying perfectly the impermanence of things.

Impermanence is one of the basic concepts of Buddhism. Everything is destined to come to an end or to change in nature one day or another. As everything is interdependent, lacking in intrinsic reality, and void, it is necessary to ground oneself in that which is without characteristics: Awakening. This is not a pessimistic concept of life but, on the contrary, a powerful antidote to illusions. Perceiving clearly the impermanence of all phenomena blossoms into a kind of consciousness that keeps the world from becoming static. That evening, the impermanence of my own life had become more than just a concept.

Beginning the next day, I drowned my disappointment over so much lost effort in the swimming pool and in the arms of two young Americans I encountered in the historic flophouse of Miss Colaço, on Janpath Lane—a guest house through which all the stars of the Beat generation filed, its poets known or unknown, its muses and vamps, as well as a good portion of those European and American dreamers caught up in the spiritual whirlwind of Berkeley, the great wave of American university protests, and the aftermath of May 1968.

At Miss Colaço's one found an incredible ethnic and cultural mix, a motley gathering totally in the thrall of Tantric fever reduced to its simplest expression: wildly liberating sexuality. Ginsberg and many of the other American poets had left their mark. The muses recited to audiences simultaneously entranced and distracted by hashish, then spent amorous nights in endless ecstasy with hairy gurus, lamas, and yogis. Black Bombay, an explosive mix of hashish from Afghanistan or Kashmir and opium, came to their aid. Everywhere you looked, you saw levitation, travels into past lives, altered consciousness, reincarnations, mad egos devoured by demons in the Tibetan rite of *tcho*, mysterious orgies in the forests, awakenings and trances, and lightning surges of kundalini, that mystical energy from the depths, represented by the figure of a serpent coiled at the base of the spinal column.

A Californian recounted how she had made love with a tiger-ascetic during the time of Buddha; an Italian poet told of his spontaneous illumination at the sight of Maharishi Mahesh Yogi crossing the Delhi airport. In this base camp of enlightenment, one learned what route to take to circumambulate Mount Kailash in secret, as well as ways of encountering the members of the secret brotherhood of the Deva Dasi, or the "servants of God," comprised of women poets, musicians, dancers, and initiates of sacred sex. They still officiated in a few temples, claimed certain people, who would then offer to give you the names. In their arms, you could attain total knowledge of that ecstasy carved in the stone of Khajuraho or Mahaballipuram.

One exchanged a Frank Zappa tape for the address of an opium den in ancient Delhi, a passport for the name of a Nepalese shaman with extraordinary powers, a night of love for the transmission of a mantra, those ritual formulas by

or nestled in the pinnacle of the Sonade temple, among sacks of grain, training myself to visualize the *mandala* of my tutelary divinity. By successive absorption and dissolution, this meditation technique allowed one, over the long term, to experience emptiness of the mind.

I evaded the Indian police, who, because of border troubles with China, reduced foreigners' stays in this region of India to three weeks.

When I was finally arrested and conducted to the state border in a military jeep, I left for Dalhousie, where Kalou Rinpoche told me he would be coming soon. I waited two months, submerging myself in my copy of the *Vijnanabhairava Tantra*. One beautiful morning, after being forewarned by a dream, I started down a long dirt road and saw coming toward me on horseback, surrounded by his monks, Kalou Rinpoche. He stopped his horse and placed his hand on my head for a few seconds. I was bathed in light.

After a grand reception in the main monastery to the sounds of trumpets and conch shells, I accompanied him up to the little mountain hermitage where he would give the final teachings of Mahamudra to five yogis. They all arrived the same day, no doubt forewarned as I had been. Some had been walking for many weeks, their long hair rolled up on their heads serving as a sanctuary for a number of jumping parasites. With their extraordinarily intense regard fixed devotedly on Kalou Rinpoche's thin silhouette, the yogis followed each inflection of his soft and vibrant voice. Like them, I was totally absorbed in the power of the transmission without understanding its sense. I was not to receive this last initiation into Tibetan Buddhism until many years later.

All the same, a trip to Nepal allowed me to bring back, along with a borrowed camera, a book, *The Tantric Sculptures of Nepal*, which Christian Bourgois had published with Rocher Editions.

On the advice of Kalou Rinpoche, very impartial in his approach to the diverse mystical paths, I was on my way to Thailand, to a monastery where a particularly interesting form of meditation was practiced. I learned to concentrate on a luminous pearl located an inch below the navel and by doing so pass through, one by one, the veils of conventional illusion. As my place of residence, the abbot had assigned to me a wonderful little temple in the middle of a luxurious garden. Also staying there were a half-dozen Japanese Zen monks who had come to be initiated into this Small Vehicle practice on the advice of their masters. The universal spirit of Kalou Rinpoche was open to the practices of different schools, and knowledge of them seemed important to him. Thus, he stood apart from the quarrels among Tibetan sects, focusing on the origins of Buddhism; Hinayana, or Small Vehicle; Ch'an; Taoism; and Indian Tantrism as well.

It is to this open-mindedness, right from the beginning of my sadhana, that I owe my recognition of the links and affiliations that exist between Tantric Shivaism, Mahamudra, *dzogchen,* and Ch'an. In the last three or four years, this relationship has become fertile ground for many researchers and academics.

Then, still following Kalou Rinpoche's recommendation, I found myself in Kyoto with a master of the Rinzai school of Zen, founded by the great master of eleventh-century Ch'an, Lin-chi. My journey ended in Honolulu, where a

Taoist master, alerted by Kalou Rinpoche, was waiting for me at the airport. This strange man, dressed in a stained, threadbare black robe, wove his turquoise Impala in and out of the traffic as if it were a matter for Lao-Tzu's black ox. From him I learned the art of circular breathing, which passes through the heart, and the posture in which the left thumb is held in the right hand, particularly stable for long meditations. When it was time to go, I got one more taste of his humor:

"When you are back in France, behind the steering wheel of your car, you must realize that you are not somewhere other than in the Tao."

His guttural laugh was lost in the hubbub, his faded robe blending into the orgy of colorful skirts, loincloths, and Bermuda shorts.

I did not forget his advice as the years passed and my practice was interrupted with dark times and doubts. Then, between 1972 and 1975, I undertook a series of journeys in the northwest of India, determined to follow leads I'd gotten on my previous trips and find a great master of Kashmirian Tantric Shivaism.

3

The next three journeys led me to discover the sublime Himalayan landscapes of Jammu, Kashmir, and Himachal Pradesh, as well as a good number of "sages," hermits, and charlatans, without a single decisive meeting taking place.

To come into direct contact with Shivaic Tantrism is nearly impossible. The first reason for this difficulty is linked to the persecutions imposed upon Tantrism by various invaders: the Aryans, the Islamics of the Middle Ages, and then the English Puritans of the colonization. The second reason is linked to the secrecy that surrounds masters and rituals.

From the time they first arrived, the invaders showed strong opposition to Tantric Shivaism, which finds its strength in being rooted in worship devoted to the Great Goddess. A warlike society cannot tolerate a culture for which the female is so central, as both origin and way of enlightenment, master and initiator. This goes against all that Puritanism and other invading forces stood for.

In Shivaism, the female embodies the power; the male, the capacity for wonder. Many of the masters were, and still are, women. Certain lineages are transmitted only through women, and, as an adept, the woman has greater credit than the man in terms of power, courage, and depth of vision. The texts clearly state: "What a male tantrika realizes in one year, a female adept attains in one day," as if, all by herself, she is naturally rooted in all that makes up the forgotten substratum that the great ancient religions have in common. From the Celts to the Dravidians of the Indus valley, from Egypt to Babylon, the basis of the human psyche is entirely woven out of the divinity of the female. The various surges of the hordes, often less barbarian than they say, and bearers of great cultural forces, skills, and knowledge that breathed new life into Hinduism and allowed the arts their marvelous flowering, never succeeded in subduing this mysterious feminine power, still alive today in Tantrism.

No moral discredit whatsoever mars the woman. Far from being the source of sin, temptation, and damnation as in the three great monotheistic religions, as well as in certain tendencies of Hinduism and Buddhism, she is, on the contrary, the power and force for transmission of the highest mystical teaching.

These feminine values, which give a unique and very contemporary air to Tantrism, can be defined briefly as deep, harmonious, and peaceful strength as opposed to violence. Spontaneity and openness as opposed to artificial moral order, hypocrisy, Puritanism. Non-duality, which restores completeness to being human by locating the divine within the self. Liberalism, tolerance, direct experience of nature fundamentally free from thought, as opposed to the vain speculations of religious sects and intellectuals. Love as opposed to sexual exploitation. Respect for nature as opposed to frenzied depletion of its resources. Absolute freedom with regard to dogmas, the clergy, the state, the caste system, and the social, religious, dietary, and sexual taboos of classical Hinduism derived from Aryan Vedism. All these values derive from unconditional respect for each human being's freedom, which Tantrism proposes to rediscover without getting lost in an external, illusory quest.

An important segment of society today realizes that we must return to these values or else suffer chaos and destruction. The Tantric way is open to all the richness of human nature, which it accepts without a single restriction. It is probably the only spiritual path that excludes nothing and no one, and, in this way, it corresponds to the deep aspirations of women and men today. Those who accept the marvelous recognition of female power and the feminine part within themselves, source of richness and continual development, no longer have a position to defend in the war between the sexes. They have integrated this recognition and gone beyond the persistent duality that impedes all deep progress.

Seven thousand years* of a continuous Tantric tradition includes an incredible art of concealment from the "foreigner." This prudence has always existed. In northern India, Tantrism is everywhere, but the closer one approaches

---

*The most ancient texts date from 5500 B.C. See Alain Danielou, *While the Gods Play* (Rochester, Vt.: Inner Traditions International, 1987).

it, the more invisible it seems. Many times I've had the sensation of being in the vicinity of a gathering place, brushing up against a master or an adept who could have guided me, but invariably the "Tantric filter" was put in place and I found myself alone, in the middle of nowhere, incapable of knowing at what point I was the victim of disinformation or of a joke—variations in a thousand-year-old protection system. After all, wasn't I myself only a new type of invader? Why should the doors be opened?

Shivaic Tantrism does not depend upon the West for its survival. Its masters still don't respond to the West's desire to import it, nor to Western curiosity, nor to its lures of profit. Tantrism is not afraid of any political power, any wave of history. The flame always flares up again; the teachings reemerge, even after the darkest periods.

One of the difficulties in encountering a master comes from the fact that traditionally Tantrism develops in the countryside, in the forests, in isolated places. Large gatherings are rare. Adepts establish themselves in the country, and the uninitiated, even if they think they know of a master, are generally afraid to pass along this information. Popular belief, with the aid of classical Hinduism, attributes to Tantric sages all sorts of evil powers and demonic practices. How could it be otherwise for a mysticism that holds the woman in such high esteem? That recognizes no castes, or any of the social, dietary, or moral taboos to which the Hindus subject themselves?

After thousands of kilometers crossed by bus, in a jeep, by foot, or on the back of ponies, after hundreds of bills handed out for food, lodging, and information, I came to the conclusion that Shivaic Tantrism would always elude me and I should give up trying to encounter one of its masters. Besides, how do you find someone whose name you don't know? In Shivaic Tantrism, to speak or write the name of one's master is forbidden. Sometimes I found myself in front of an abandoned hut, an empty cave, or a village idiot who had been pointed out to me as a sage and who could very well have been one. I would understand much later that the appearance of the fool is one of the tantrikas' favorite disguises.

Then, on my fourth journey, after several fruitless attempts, I decided to abandon my quest, to forget about my Bartholomew map covered with red circles and mysterious routes. I could no longer continue accosting the faithful who, at dawn, went to leave an offering or a bouquet of flowers at the black stone *linga* (phallus) of Shiva, symbolizing the destruction of illusion, erected on a pedestal in the form of a vulva, or *yoni*, emblem of mysterious cosmic power. I could no longer follow the steep paths of the naked ascetics smeared with ashes, and risk having myself impaled on their iron tridents, sign of Shiva and symbol of the subtle channels that cross the yogis' bodies. I had no more money to pay "informers," my feet couldn't bear any more blisters, and I'd had enough of finding myself once again, come evening, in a clearing or under a new moon where a Tantric ritual was supposed to take place. When I asked any questions about Tantrism, nearly always the response was "What?" as if it were a matter of the latest advance in physics.

From Manali to Sonarmarg, Himalayan routes and paths held no more secrets for me. The last Shivaic master was supposed to live at the summit of Mount Kailash, the very place where Shiva had reappeared to give the secret teachings to the people of the Kali Yuga, or the dark age, of which I had not seen the beginning (about 3600 B.C.) and would not see the end (about A.D. 2440). Nevertheless, the sages say that Tantrism corresponds exactly to the needs, capacities, and hopes of the beings of this period.

One day the bus stopped. Two women got off, one of them carrying a rooster by the legs. There was no village in sight. Without even thinking, I shouted to the driver to open the door again. Not a minute longer did I want to be on this bus with all its bolts rattling, as, under the apparent control of its Sikh driver, it hurtled down the slopes of the Himalayan foothills at breakneck speed. Once the bus departed, I found myself in a refreshing silence. The women climbed a path and chatted, the rooster protesting. I followed them. There had to be a village up there.

Half an hour later, I arrived at it. About thirty earth houses were spread out over a large plateau. A river meandered nearby. This seemed to me the ideal place to rest and forget about Tantrism. An adolescent approached me; I knew right away that I should trust him.

"Hello Sahib; my name is Ram. Can I help you?"

I asked him to find a house for me to rent for several weeks. He tracked one down for me, at the edge of the village, near a splendid banyan tree at the foot of which I discovered several signs of Shiva: his *linga* firmly embedded in the *yoni* of his Shakti; a small bull, Nandi, their favorite medium; and several garlands of flowers as well as some pastries. One of them was decorated with a fine coat of pure silver that the air made quiver. A village woman paid me a visit. The cottage suited me perfectly. A *charpoy,* a wood box tied with cord, a small hearth on the hard-packed earthen floor, a corner for washing. Twenty square meters of perfection. I was asked for thirty rupees for the month, and, as soon as the transaction was completed, a blanket, a jug of potable water, an armful of wood, a bowl of yogurt, four potatoes, an onion, a tea bag, a saucepan, a little oil, some matches, salt, and a kettle were brought in, with the discreet efficiency you find throughout India as soon as you leave the beaten paths.

As all the village children came by, one by one, to stick their heads in the doorway, Ram helped me light a fire and watched, fascinated, as I opened my backpack. I put my sleeping bag on the *charpoy*, my many books and my note-book near the bed. I offered him a tin box of Indian cheese, and he took me visiting in the village, proud to present me to the doctor and his wife as well as to the other inhabitants, who regarded me with astonishment. What could a stranger be coming here to find?

After briefly summarizing my life to about twenty of the curious, I answered the urgent, charming questions of those lively, gracious children and adolescents. Then I returned to the calm of my little house. Ram sold tea with milk and ginger root in delicate little goblets of sun-dried earth that were thrown away after use, their crumbling material re-turned to the ground. Each morning, Ram brought new goblets. Thus we took up the habit, come daybreak, of warming ourselves by his fire, drinking and watching the frail silhouettes, draped in shawls, leave the fog rising off the river, and come, shivering, to search out Ram's ener-gizing brew. I felt relieved at having abandoned my quest, and I used my morning wake-up ritual for meditating, wrapped in my blanket, before going to drink tea, taking along a few coals for Ram's fire. With great dignity, the youth made use of a large sieve in which could be found all the tea served since daybreak. For each new client, he added a pinch of fresh tea.

I forgot about Tantrism so well that I spent a good part of my days walking along the river and in the forest, often accompanied by Ram, hand in hand, as is the Indian custom. Sometimes I was accompanied by the other adolescents with their large, dark eyes and long black hair. Delicate, dignified, free, and modest at the same time, they stretched toward the sky in that very beautiful posture that comes from habitually carrying jars and packages on one's head.

Ram had a friendly nature. He was curious and lively, and knew everything despite his young age. A deep friendship grew between us, nourished by his vision of life and his hopes, desires, and fears. He absorbed information with remarkable intelligence and already possessed that calm attitude toward things that comes only with time. One by one, he helped me get to know all the inhabitants of the village, where I could soon go from one house to another as though I'd been born there.

Sometimes, in the evening, I would go to talk with the doctor who owned the only stone house in the village. Retired for a few years, he practiced ayurvedic medicine and continued to treat the villagers.

I learned how to make yogurt. My proximity to the banyan tree and the Shiva where delicacies were left sometimes let me take advantage of those offerings deposited by women in sumptuous saris, their strong vibrant colors shimmering in the morning light. The smell of incense entered the cottage. I went to bathe in the icy water of the river. I read and reread the *Vijnanabhairava Tantra* and practiced assiduously and regularly to the point of reaching that state again that I had known at the end of my first year of continuous practice—that state in which one desires only one thing: to remain in meditation for hours, unmoving, as if fixed in the center of space; full of warmth, energy, openness; breathing deeply, regularly, and silently— the mandala, constructing itself before you as if projected, each detail intensely present, the mantra flowing like a river, the phases of absorption following from one another smoothly until the final void.

I used this particularly beneficial period for practicing guru yoga and for visualizing Vajradhara, the Tibetan divinity who represents the spiritual master and whose blue body appeared effortlessly, framed in empty space, facing me. For the first time, I succeeded in practicing dream yoga regularly. This form of yoga allows one to become conscious of dreams and to enter meditation, thus replacing the dream with the mandala or directly with non-dualistic contemplation. When I awakened, this meditation left a sensation of great freshness, of deep rest free of the anarchic activities of consciousness; the mind was lucid and open.

Soon I was laughing at my frenzied Tantric quest and tasting the simple pleasure of *being* in this lost village, of walking and of meditating in total tranquility. Kalou Rinpoche had often spoken to me of the peace that comes with abandoning effort, tension, and the desire to attain something. Now I experienced it daily. Each act of living—rising, drinking a cup or two of tea, eating a little, following the course of the turquoise water, entering the forest, reading a sutra, walking hand in hand with a happy youth under the starry sky—brought me incomparable joy.

One day, following the river upstream for a few hours, I came to a sort of basin, very deep, with a waterfall four or five meters high. The spot, strewn with large rock polished by the river's high waters, was wonderfully peaceful. All alone, I burst out laughing and took a swim in the deeper, darker water of the basin before drying myself on a warm stone. The place was dominated by a twelve-meter cliff and a thick forest. I fell asleep in the sun. When I awoke, I had the strange sensation of being watched. I looked all around and listened without seeing a living soul.

One couldn't reach the top of the cliff directly without going back down the river to a steep trail with a difficult access. I decided to climb up to explore the edge of the forest.

Once there, I discovered a hillock from which I could enjoy a splendid view of the river, the waterfall, and the neighboring hills, which were almost lost in the golden light. I took a few steps into the forest, and there I discovered a hut, a bed of grass, a hearth with warm cinders, a terracotta pot, a few white garments, a faded blanket, some blackened cooking utensils, and a bowl made from the top of a human skull, its rim set with silver. All of a sudden, I imagined an ascetic threatening me with his trident, and I hurried out of there.

All the way back, my imagination was in a state of agitation far from meditative. I ran the last hundred meters, impatient to talk to Ram about my discovery. He was waiting for me, peacefully seated on the stone-lined pedestal of the banyan.

I told him about my excursion and his face darkened.

"Don't ever go back to the waterfall! That woman is very dangerous! She killed a man last year. They fished his body out of the river. She eats the dead. She is a tantrika!"

4

I slept very little that night, haunted by the idea that a Tantric yogini was living nearby, a few hours away by foot. The description that Ram had given me was hardly encouraging. I thought about the man found dead in the river. The fact that Ram described her as a devourer of dead bodies impressed me less, that being a cliche often found in Tantric literature. I imagined a thousand ways of approaching her, of trying to see her, and of convincing her to accept me as a disciple.

I was the first one under the banyan. Ram came to light his fire, and while he warmed the water and the milk I bombarded him with questions about the yogini.

"How long has she been living near the waterfall?"

"A little over a year."

"Have you ever seen her?"

"She is a monster. The eyes of a crazy person, a huge red tongue that hangs out of her mouth, drops of dried blood on her belly, hair all disheveled. Some of the villagers have seen her. At night she walks through the forest with a big knife and kills animals to drink their blood. No one goes to the waterfall anymore since she moved there. It's very dangerous!"

Ram tried to imitate her by making a horrible face and sticking out his tongue.

"Is she Indian?"

"No, she's a sorceress from Tibet who came down out of the mountains."

"Nobody goes to visit her?"

"Sometimes some yogis come through the village. We think they're going to the waterfall."

"Tibetans?"

"No, only Indians."

"Then she must be Indian."

During this whole conversation, Ram avoided looking at me. I sensed that he was tense, irritated, and distant. He remained silent for a moment and prepared two cups of tea, dark and fragrant. While we drank the piping hot liquid in little sips, he said to me:

"If you are my friend, you must trust me. If you go up there, you will never return. She will kill you. She will eat your liver and your heart. The rest of you will go to feed the fish. You will have paid to rent this house and you won't be in it anymore. I won't come to find you. If you want to meet a guru, there's one near Srinagar. He's famous. He has a beautiful ashram; people come from all over the world to see him. He is a very good old man. If you want me to, I'll take you there. Ask the doctor, he knows. Do you want to take the next bus?"

"No. I want to stay here, to see this monster of the waterfall from a distance. If she looks the way you say she does, I'll come back down."

"You aren't the first one to want to meet her. The danger is that she can make herself invisible, and when you get to the waterfall, she can kill you before you even have time to grab a rock."

I finished another cup of ginger tea, and, not very convinced by Ram's descriptions, I decided to use this clear morning to climb to the waterfall. I debated over what to take. I didn't know whether I would succeed in seeing her, much less in talking to her. After a few minute's reflection, I put my sleeping bag, some tea, a few provisions, the blanket I'd been lent, and my knife into my pack. Passing by the banyan tree again, I waved to Ram, who didn't respond. I took a garland of flowers given to Shiva as an offering to his Shakti, and I was on my way.

With each step I tried to uproot the childish images that Ram had planted in my mind. Nevertheless, the fact that they had found a dead man in the river made an impression on me. I had approached enough nagas and Shivaic ascetics to know that they could be violent. Even the Indian police gave up arresting them because their total indifference to prison and their magical powers spread uncontrollable terror among the other inmates and sparked revolts. Nothing could stop these ascetics, and many Western journalists who tried to film them had had a hard time of it. I remembered that a few of them had been tossed into the Yamuna or thrown from a mirador at the Kumbha-Mela, one of the great religious gatherings, which sometimes assembles more than a million Indians of all persuasions.

As soon as I regained the silence of the mountain, my fear seemed to rise, like dough exposed to warmth. Each attempt to reassure myself had the opposite effect. More than once I asked myself whether I should turn around and go back.

My curiosity was stronger, and toward ten o'clock I heard the noise of the waterfall. I sat down and tried to work out a method of approach. If I climbed directly to the hermitage, I stood a chance of finding the yogini in her hut, but I also ran the risk of disturbing her and being very badly received. If I went for a swim, alerting her, as it were, of my presence without imposing, I ran the risk of no longer finding her by climbing up to the hermitage.

I opted for a third solution: I approached within a hundred meters of the hut, left my offerings of food and the garland, made three great prostrations in the Tibetan style, and retreated toward the waterfall, where I found a flat rock for meditation. I wanted her to understand that I was not motivated by curiosity, to show her evidence of my respect, and to give her the opportunity to summon me in one way or another.

Despite the stability of the posture, I had much difficulty in finding tranquility. I meditated for two or three hours, swam, dried myself in the sun, and took up my meditation again. At no time did I have the sensation of being observed, as opposed to the first time. I stopped meditating toward the end of the afternoon. I was hungry, and realized that I'd offered all my provision to the Shakti. I was dying to know whether my offerings had been accepted, and I climbed back up toward the esplanade.

Once there, I saw to my great disappointment that

everything was still where I had left it. I could barely make out the hut, hidden by some trees, but I imagined that if the yogini was in there, she could see me. I made three more prostrations and headed back toward the village. About halfway, much to my surprise, I saw a very anxious Ram waiting for me. Moved by his affection, I took him by the hand and we went back down toward the familiar landscape of little houses, colorful saris, mouth-watering smells, and the cries of children.

"If you truly wish to see her, you must offer milk, ginger, rice, good tea, lentils, eggs, spices, incense, and a very beautiful garland of flowers. Give me twelve rupees and I will find you all that for tomorrow," said Ram, who understood that I would not be discouraged.

We ate dinner together and I went to bed early, ready to leave at daybreak loaded up with offerings.

I climbed more quickly and arrived in good time on the esplanade, where I noted with satisfaction that my presents of the day before had vanished. I then deposited Ram's various things, prostrated myself, and went back to meditate on my rock. The journey had been more peaceful, and my meditation was more profound, my mind more relaxed.

I waited until the last hour to return to the village and found Ram waiting for me in the same spot. He began to take part in my quest and stamped his feet with impatience because he had left out something. Again I gave him some ten-rupee notes with which he bought some matches, candles, and a pure wool shawl. I admired the methodical manner in which he foresaw the needs of a solitary ascetic, and I put my entire trust in him.

This time again, the presents had been accepted. At the moment when I was about to leave the garland of flowers and my offerings, I saw the yogini standing at the edge of the forest. She wore light clothes: jodhpurs and a tunic. Her long black hair was not tied up. Her facial characteristics I couldn't see clearly because of the distance. I felt my heart beating violently; I made three prostrations and approached. She remained immobile. Her face slowly became visible, and I saw no enormous tongue, no bloodstains, no wild, bulging eyes. To the contrary, I found her bearing free of flaws, open, beautiful, and noble.

As I stood before her she held me in her extraordinarily brilliant regard. She had to be about forty years old but showed little mark of the ascetic life. She was simultaneously light and powerful, close and distant. She wore a red necklace decorated with small bells. Her look emanated immense compassion, which her physical bearing, more reserved, seemed to temper. I was astonished when she addressed me in perfect English.

"Where do you come from? What are you looking for?"

"From France . . . I'm looking for someone who can open me up to the understanding and the practice of Shivaism, of kundalini yoga."

"I don't know kundalini yoga."

"Aren't you a tantrika?"

"What do you know about Tantrism?"

"A few years ago, a Chinese yogi gave me a copy of his translation of the *Vijnabhairava Tantra*. I've read it often. I even have it here with me."

"Show it to me."

I took it out of the top pocket of my pack, where I kept

notes and books. She flipped through it quickly, then gave it back.

"The Chinese yogi is an impostor. This is not the *Vijnanabhairava Tantra*. But you haven't answered me. What do you know about Tantrism?"

"I assume that in Tantrism there is a practice that leads to entering into harmony with one's own heart and discovering Shiva there."

"Tantrism contains none of this kind of sentimentalism."

"And the sexual practices, do they exist?"

"If there were sexual practices in Tantrism, how could I devote myself to it, since I've lived alone for sixteen years?"

"Perhaps by transcending them?"

"There is nothing to transcend in Tantrism."

Suddenly, my mind stopped wandering. I felt myself melting under her regard, and tears came to my eyes.

"I would like to follow your teaching."

"Your emotions don't concern me. You have an idea of what it is you're looking for. How can you find it? I can give you nothing. Return to the valley."

I took leave of the yogini in a state of intense emotion, stripped naked by her look. I picked up my pack and took a few steps backward. As I was turning around she spoke to me in a gentler voice, with an indescribable smile.

"You are like a hunchback in the country. You imagine that by leaving the town, no one will see your hump. Forget how others regard you and truly consider your hump. It is the most precious thing you have."

On my way back down to the village, I was torn between the impression of complete failure and the hope of a possible opening.

When Ram saw me arrive, he understood immediately that something had taken place. Also, he greeted me, laughing:

"You walk like an old man!"

I straightened up, drank a few cups of tea, and gave him an account of my adventure, savoring the delicious potato fritters with curry and mustard seeds that his mother had prepared for us.

I spent the days that followed caressing my hump and realized that I could only present myself before the yogini completely naked, without desires and without goals.

Each morning, I made offerings to the Shiva *linga* found at the foot of the banyan, hoping that this stone phallus would end up embedding itself in my heart and open it to the dimensions of space.

5

When I went back up to the hermitage with a simple garland as an offering, I felt full of confidence and joy. I found the yogini meditating in front of her hut. I made a simple Indian salute, holding my palms before my heart like a lotus ready to open, and sat down quite a distance away from her. Her eyes were half closed. Grace, beauty, and power emanated from her entire being, as if the long years of solitary practice had planted her in the ground, and her deep rooting allowed branches to spread out harmoniously into space.

She opened her eyes. I greeted her again and approached, holding out the garland of flowers, which she hung around her neck.

"That's all that you brought me today?" she said ironically.

After a few awkward moments, I bowed again, as if to tell her: I bring my hump, I bring my heart. But I remained silent because that seemed to me both naive and grandiloquent.

"I will accept you on the condition that you reflect deeply upon what I am going to tell you and that you take the time to decide whether you want to follow this quest," she said, as if she had heard me.

Full of joy, I thanked her.

"Understand that this is a very deep commitment on my part and on yours. Once on the way, there is no exit. If you accept, it's a decision that must be maintained in the most difficult moments, because if you give up along the way, you risk deep trouble. I am proposing that you make your way along a razor's edge. Once you start out, you can't break into a run, or stop, or go back. The injuries would be very serious. You can only continue at the same pace. Sometimes you will revolt. You will have the impression that I'm treating you as if you've never practiced, as if you know nothing. Your pride will be hurt. You will think, I did this, I did that. I have had so-and-so a master, and this woman, who is she to treat me like this? You will have doubts about yourself, about the way, about me. You will be angry. Perhaps you will hate me. But me, I will always be there and I will wait for you to calm yourself so that we can get under way again together. What is your name?"

"Karma."

"In Tantrism, *karma* is considered illusory, but I will call you Karma."

"What should I call you?"

"Sometimes I am Kali, the destroyer, sometimes I am Lalita, the playful one, sometimes I am Kubjika, the potter, but I am always Devi, the goddess. So call me Devi. At first, when you came, you made great prostrations. Today, you greeted me in the Indian style. When you do that, what image comes to mind?"

"One of devotion, of respect, the hope of receiving and realizing the most precious teachings."

"Do you think there's a fundamental difference between you and me?"

"Yes, you are a master."

"When you greet me, do not bow before someone who may be what you are not. Even if Shiva were standing there in front of you, never bow before something distant and unattainable; on the contrary, bow before that which links us and which makes us fundamentally alike, which makes Shiva and his companion, Bhairavi, fundamentally no different from you and me. When you bow, bow deeply before the divine which is in ourselves and in this moment, before the divine which has never been separate from us, before the divine which is not found anywhere other than in ourselves, before the divine which one can never get closer to or farther away from, before the inconceivable divine out of which our entire being is fashioned, as the texture of clay out of which we take the form given to us by the potter. As long as you imagine a way which separates you from the divine, you are preparing for lengthy wandering, and this wandering will never end, because the more you think you are approaching the divine, the more it will escape you.

"Shiva is inconceivable, unattainable, and yet it is impossible to distance yourself from him, because fundamentally you are Shiva. You greet me, you greet the divine which links us like the ground on which we both walk, like the sky in which our gaze gets lost."

Devi paused for a long silence. She looked at me as if her words were taking time to penetrate my consciousness. She spoke slowly and deliberately, in a soft voice, as one would tell a story to a child. I looked at her and realized suddenly that a very long route had brought me exactly here. I thought of the razor image she had used and asked myself whether I would have the courage to follow this teaching. I could not imagine how she could trigger the reactions of doubt, rejection, and hate in me that she predicted. I thought suddenly of Kalou Rinpoche, who had, until now, bestowed his teachings upon me without subjecting me to terrible tests. It is true that Westerners are often impatient in their quests and that Kalou Rinpoche had taught me patience. I'd watched many Westerners arrive and, after spending three or four days at the monastery, go off in search of less time-consuming teachings. Devi took up again with the same calm voice:

"In Tantrism, fundamentally there is no temple, no God, no dogmas, no beliefs. There is only an immense umbilical cord, which reunites each being and each thing in the divine. To experience an awakening is to glimpse that in its totality, even in the space of a second. To experience Great Awakening is to evolve continually in this single infinite space that consciousness is wed to when Shiva and Bhairavi become one, when the ecstasy of their union overflows into the consciousness, opened so wide it can no longer even say, 'I am the consciousness, I am the limitless, I am the totality of the divine.'

"Consciousness is the place of worship. Consciousness is the sacred text. Consciousness is the way. Consciousness is the place of sacrifice. Consciousness is the fire. Consciousness is the place of ritual union. Consciousness is the place of *samadhi*. Consciousness is the Awakening. Consciousness is the dwelling place of the gods. Consciousness is time. Consciousness is space. Consciousness is the jar, the vessel out of which flows the divine.

"What does the worshiper do? He cleans the temple. How? By asking all who have been sitting there forever to leave so he can sweep, throw fresh water drawn from the river on the stones, scatter rose petals. Very quickly, the worshiper takes count of those sitting in his consciousness who refuse to leave the temple. Why? Because, like us, they are afraid. It is because of fear that the consciousness remains cluttered. Not the little fears, easy to define, not the fear of this or that, but the great fundamental fear, which is the fragile terrain on which we construct all our dreams, and which, one day or another, paralyzes us and destroys what we have constructed with so much care.

"The day to act arrives. You purify yourself by bathing in the sacred river. You feel alive and full of determination. You draw fresh water, take a broom, gather a basket of rose petals, and enter the temple of the consciousness. That is meditation: to enter fresh, the mind alive and alert in the temple of the consciousness. You see them, all seated, immobile, anchored in the ground, fossilized. They have been there for such a long time. They have loved you so much, given you so much, spared you so much. Since you were very young, their voices have guided you. Even now, at this moment, as they watch you enter, ready to clean, freshen, and scent, they talk to you and you listen: 'Listen, this is what we think of you. Since you were young, we've been trying to keep you from danger, to warn you of life's pitfalls. We punish you when you make a mistake, but when you listen to us, when you are a good boy, we reward you, we sing your praises, and, thanks to us, you haven't come out too badly. Now then, don't chase us away. Keep listening to our voices, following our advice. We only want what's best for you. Freedom? It's chaos. Listen to us closely, follow the way we show you, and all will go well.'

"But in this instant, you know that you have listened too much, that these stone-colored men are there only to keep you from scattering the roses and the fresh water. That all is not going so well. You are like two fears face-to-face. Like two fears finding themselves nose-to-nose in a dark forest, full of creaking and cracking and other frightening sounds. One fear says to itself, 'Let's hope that he doesn't do anything to eject us from the temple!' The other fear says to itself, 'Let's hope they don't get up to go out! What would become of me without them!' And like that, day after day, one compromises with the consciousness, receives blame and encouragement, falls into line, and becomes someone for whom grayness is acceptable. All of society adores the monochrome of gray. Gray is the most widespread color. There are millions of varieties. Gray is the ideal color for social camouflage. It is thanks to our gray that we manage to exist socially, to merge into the immense cauldron of suffering and ordinary violence."

Devi sensed that this suffering, this "ordinary" violence, elicited strong feelings in me. She fell silent and gave me a probing look. Letting the thread of my thought unwind, she seemed to touch each loop. I had the impression that she listened into my silence. This suffering and violence were the reasons for my being here. I wanted to try to put an end to them without always shifting responsibility onto others, without always wanting *the others* to stop being violent. Devi placed me before my own responsibility. What part of my consciousness served as a vital link to suffering and violence? How was I myself also a machine of destruction? How was the body, that huge battlefield of cells, a prefiguration for the world? How could I attain a practice that could begin to change the world, starting with the only thing directly accessible: my own consciousness of reality? Devi started to answer me:

"In Tantrism, there is fundamentally only one color: red. The color of the living heart, the color of blood, the color of fire, the color of roses and of the tongue, the color of the open vulva, the color of the erect penis, the color of the sun that warms the hermits, the color of the circle of fire that must be crossed to attain consciousness. Shiva comes from the root *Shiv,* which means 'red' in Tamil.

"The first thing a tantrika does is conquer this fear. He lets out a great cry, a cry of rebirth, and drives all those little gray men out of the consciousness. It is very difficult. It takes much courage to spread fresh water and rose petals on the empty stones of the temple. One has only one desire: to run after the gray men and ask them humbly to come back. Besides, for a long time, they wait outside the temple. They stay within earshot. They watch for a moment of weakness on your part.

"For a few seconds, you feel very much alone, abandoned by everyone. Space is too big and too empty. You tremble. You have trouble throwing out everything that the little gray men have left behind, as if to claim their territory. You have trouble getting the water to rinse over the stones. But as soon as you've washed them down, as soon as you've thrown the petals, you feel a great freshness—a divine, fragrant, completely open space. This is your own empty consciousness.

"Then comes the most difficult moment, much more difficult even than abandoning your fear. When the temple is empty and resplendent, so that the light shimmers in it, the songs of the birds fill it, fragrances scent it, and moonbeams make it even more spacious, we congratulate ourselves for our wisdom and clear-sightedness, and we say to ourselves, 'Now this place is absolutely pure. It's the perfect spot for storing the sublime teachings I've had access to. In this temple, I'm going to store the most profound products of wisdom to nourish my consciousness.'

"At first, you feel wonderfully well. You introduce great and beautiful notions, a pure ideal, brilliant teachings. The whole universe seems glad to take part in your plan. Little by little, you build yourself a very beautiful world theory, and you perfect your knowledge. Nevertheless, things gradually and imperceptibly change. At first you don't notice. You cling to the idea that there is only the sublime in the temple; nevertheless, already you don't feel completely at ease there any longer, especially since you want to see others conform to this dearly won *truth*. Already you begin to exercise violence against others and yourselves.

"One night, in your sleep, you believe you hear a voice, then two, then ten or twenty, and in the morning when you wake up, you see that all the little gray men are back in the temple. You listen to their whispering, quiet at first, then more and more obtrusive. To gain entry, they've watched for opportunities to attach themselves to the notions and beliefs you've allowed into the empty temple."

I felt myself disarmed by Devi's capacity to restore to me my own responsibility, by her spiral-like way of teaching, during the course of which all my questions found answers.

"Now, go back to your place. If you truly want to wash out the temple, return when you are ready. Return with enough provisions for a long period of time, put your affairs in order, and I will teach you the way of Tantrism."

Profoundly moved, I bowed before the divine in us, but this was still only an idea. I didn't really feel the umbilical cord she'd spoken about.

"Don't forget the rose petals," Devi said.

I went back up to the hermitage supplied with rice, rolled oats, barley flour, cheese, salt, and sugar. I brought my kerosene stove, my cooking utensils, books, sleeping bag, and the blanket I'd been lent.

Devi, wrapped in her light wool shawl, was walking along the edge of the forest. She seemed to be looking for something. I put down my pack and greeted her, and she returned my greeting. She was gay and playful this morning. When she laughed, she took on the air of a carefree adolescent. Already I was astonished by her capacity to change, and I still knew only one or two of her infinite forms.

"This is where you'll build your hut. You will be fine here, sheltered from the wind and near the waterfall and the spring where we draw water. When you've finished, rest, go down to bathe, and bring some stones back up to make your hearth. Then come see me in my hut."

Once Devi left, I prepared the ground, then went deeper

into the forest to find the necessary building materials. My knife was sharp enough to serve as a hatchet. I built a cabin of branches with a pitched roof. It measured about two meters long by one and a half meters wide. In this season, I didn't need to worry about rain, and I counted on facing the cool nights equipped with my sleeping bag designed for the Himalayan cold. The temperature, very pleasant during the day, dropped rapidly after sunset. It took me seven or eight hours to build this makeshift shelter, which opened onto the esplanade. My hut was situated fifty meters away from Devi's.

When that was finished, I inflated my sleeping pad and arranged my bed, blanket, books, and the small treasures at the bottom of my pack: candles, matches, lighter, extra kerosene, and a new wick for the stove, necessary for cooking. To be economical I had decided to use the stove for tea and breakfast, and build myself a fire to prepare the other meals.

It was only when I arrived at the great basin of green water and plunged in that I realized what had happened to me. I had taken the step. There I was, cut off from the world. I started to tremble, not because of the cold water but because of my fundamental fear, which I still had only begun to grasp. As the sun sank, I dried myself quickly, dressed, and struggled back up with the stones, which were to retain a heat more lasting than the coals.

When I arrived at Devi's hut, she told me to enter. The burning fire radiated a gentle warmth. Sitting on an old blanket folded in quarters, she asked me to go find mine and to take a place facing her.

Once I was situated, she looked at me for a long time. Lit up by the flames, her dark, terribly brilliant eyes gave me the impression of a fountain of love pouring toward me. Her look also had something of the power of a fire in the forest, which drives away all the imagined forms that never stop appearing to us. She opened one of her hands and there I saw some small pebbles, which she must have collected at the river. Near me was a pot. By throwing in a stone, she made it ring. I smiled because her aim was perfect.

"This pot represents your mind. Each time you cease to be here by taking refuge in your thoughts, I will throw a little stone. Thus you will become aware of the number of disturbances you create to escape from the present reality. When we look at each other, Shiva and Shakti look at each other. Why are Shiva and Shakti divine? Because nothing comes to disrupt them from being present with each other. To be Shiva isn't difficult. It's enough to be present, to be entirely there, moment after moment. If you only realized this one Tantric teaching, you would attain the divine. You would be an integral part of the divine, which you enjoy imagining in me but which you still don't recognize in yourself. No asceticism leads to a distant divinity. All we imagine elsewhere is in ourselves. To be Shiva is to realize that spontaneously. Are you ready to wash down the temple?"

"Yes. I've thought about the conditions you've laid out. I agree to go to the very end."

Devi laughed.

"That's very courageous on your part. I have visited your hut. It's built well. Follow my teachings in the same manner."

I thanked her for accepting me as a disciple. Then she asked me a question, which totally threw me.

"Tell me about your first experience of awakening."

"If I am here, it's precisely because I haven't had any awakening experience."

"If you haven't had any experience of awakening, I can't do anything for you."

She let my confusion increase. Then she began again.

"Without prior experience of awakening, no asceticism, no practice, no meditation bears fruit. Without awakening experience, there is no source, and since all Tantric *sadhana* consist of returning to the source, one wanders, not knowing where to go. You could follow my teachings for thirty years. Without prior awakening experience, you'd arrive at nothing. Look into yourself deeply. Think about your childhood, your adolescence. An awakening experience is found there. No being exists on earth who hasn't had this fundamental experience."

Devi stood up and put her right hand on my head. I felt a wonderful sort of light and warmth, and suddenly an image appeared.

"I was eleven years old. I was on vacation in the mountains. I had met a young girl my age, and one evening we went out along a path that rose above the village. We held hands and walked in silence. At one moment, we stopped and looked at the sky. The incredibly luminous stars seemed closer. I had the impression of being totally dissolved into the sky. It lasted a few seconds. Could that be called an awakening?"

"When no sensation of the ego remains, nor of duality, nor of the mental operation that makes us say 'How beautiful it is, how infinite!'—when there's nothing to limit an experience, when the mind rediscovers space, then it's a matter of awakening. From now on, you are no longer on a search for an abstract or remote state. You're searching for nothing that is not already within you. This capacity for total wonder is the very substance of awakening. It is out of this and only this that you become a man. All the other quests, all the other pleasures, are evasions."

"But I thought that there was Awakening, with a capital A, and only with that would come deliverance, the end of illusion."

"Between the awakening you know and the awakening I know, there's only one difference. That's duration. And when you realize that time doesn't exist, how can your awakening take refuge in a limited span of time?"

"There's no difference in intensity?"

"None. The intensity comes precisely from the fact that there's no end to it. There's no return to restrictive activity. All activity, all play of the mind takes place within Awakening. Everything can enter and leave, everything can emerge, everything can be tasted in all its richness."

"But why do we lose this capacity for wonder?"

"Because the little gray men come to reside in the consciousness. Education, society, sick love, hate, desire, jealousy, ambition, mental and material quests—all these things make us strangers to ourselves. We think only of copying, imitating, achieving new states, and whether or not our desires are fulfilled, we lose the happiness within us. Then we come to imagine heaven and hell separate from ourselves. This is a great subterfuge, which allows our consciousness to function outside of ecstasy. If man knew that he himself was God and heaven and hell, no illusions would have a hold on him; nothing could limit his consciousness.

Placing heaven outside self allows suffering to become an institution maintained by society's dream at such a high level that we can no longer escape from it. Whatever our fortune starting out in life, a day comes when we decide to limit our consciousness, to dry it up.

"As for the mystical crises of adolescence, the great revolts that make us doubt the path indicated by others, one day we step back and decide to pay our imaginary debt to society. We accept the death of our true selves. And the great fraud is that this death troubles no one. To the contrary, it is watched for, welcomed, and rewarded. As soon as the price of this spiritual death is accepted, it becomes extremely hard to follow another route. That can happen only at the cost of immense effort and very great courage. Those who have accepted their own deaths have only one possibility: to become followers of a religion or group that places the divine outside the self. Thus, everything is subsumed by society's order and interests, aligned to those of the churches and sects, which operate from the same common base: the death of divine consciousness. The driving forces are guilt, fear, obedience. The results are rigidity, distance from sensory objects, obsession, Puritanism, violence, moral codes, exclusion. In India, America, China, the Mideast, Europe—that is the mode of operation we see at work throughout.

"To become a tantrika is only to realize the fundamentally pure and heavenly nature of consciousness and to let it take over your life. When that happens, no social game, no drug, no limited ideal can become inscribed in the consciousness, but above all, no activity in the world is capable of taking away this radiance. The tantrika can then live within society and remain an unalterable diamond."

"Are there many successive awakenings before the Great Awakening?"

"If you think a Great Awakening exists, you're caught in a formidable trap, which will make you confuse an awakening with that final state. You'll remain blocked by mistaking it for what it's not. The basis of Tantric *sadhana* is always to wait for a new veil to be torn away without your spiritual qualities hardening. In nature, nothing ceases to evolve, to be infinitely transformed. To look for a stable state is to cut yourself off from reality. Everything is based on respiration. Can you breathe in for three hours? No. You breathe in and breathe out. We follow the movement of the universe, going in and out, opening and closing, expanding and contracting. All activity takes place in these two modes, and it is their perfect comprehension, their perfect integration into our practice, that allows consciousness to breathe. Never forget that consciousness breathes."

"You spoke of our fortunes starting out in life. What was it you wanted to say?"

"To be conceived through love is good fortune. To be born to a loving woman is good fortune. To be born to a yogini is good fortune. To live in a harmonious family, to meet a friend, then a spiritual master is good fortune. To have self-confidence is good fortune. To have the strength to revolt is good fortune. To cling to nothing, no philosophy, no belief, no dogma is good fortune. To remember an instance of awakening and return to this source is good fortune. To know any single one of these things is good fortune."

Devi poured two cups of fresh water and held one out to

me. I took it, and as I was going to drink I saw my face reflected in it. I stopped for a second. An idea sprang up. I heard a stone fall into the pot. I drank. Never had a cup of water seemed so wonderful to me.

"I hand you a cup of fresh water. The water seems delicious to you if you are here, tasteless if you are lost in thought. You are here, facing me, and you are happy because you think you are drinking at my spring. One needs only a bowl of really fresh water to taste its unique flavor, but if you practice drinking from someone else's spring, you will never become a fountain. To awaken is to become a fountain for others and never stop flowing. Sometimes offering a bowl of fresh water is enough to change a life. What were you thinking looking into the water?"

"I believe I began to think of the void, but the stone made the pot ring. In the past I thought about the void all the time. I was obsessed by it. It is the thing in Buddhism that seems to me the most difficult to grasp. I go around and around the void as if it were a great mystery."

"Before becoming a tantrika, I was in love with the idea of the void myself. My father was a potter, and from early childhood I'd been fascinated by his hands, which rode the clay around the void and fashioned wonderful objects out of emptiness. During adolescence I wanted to be a potter, but because of my excellent grades, my teachers told my parents that I would become a teacher. For them, that represented an important rise in social status. From that time on, my father forbade me to help him. He placed much of his hope in me. One day, I became a teacher. I was married to a teacher, and a little while after my marriage, at a market, I saw a woman my mother's age who was selling her jars, her pots, her cups. Her hands were marked by the work, and without knowing why, I approached her and I touched them. I felt the great softness that clay gives to the skin, and I began to cry. The woman comforted me in her arms. Immediately, I made my decision. I went home. I told my husband that I was leaving. He beat me very brutally, and as soon as he left the house, I withdrew my savings from the bank and I fled. I established myself in a village where there wasn't any potter, and I began to make pots and jars, thinking all the time of the wonderful void that contained my consciousness and my wonderful consciousness that contained the void. I came to understand little by little that the void was full, that fullness was empty, that the void was rooted in the clay, and that if the clay did not recognize the void, it could never become a pot or a jar. I lived very happily until one day when a tantrika came to buy a jar for his master. I told him that I wanted to take this jar back to his master myself as a present, as a testimony of what constituted my freedom. We took a bus, and then we walked in the mountains for a long time.

The master, amused, asked me if the inside of the jar was empty or full. I answered that it was full of emptiness. Immediately, he took me on as a disciple. The void no longer obsessed me. I had realized that the void is the bone and the marrow of each being, of each thing. Without the void, nothing would be possible. If you read the *Vijnanabhairava Tantra* well, you'll understand that all it talks about is the void.

Devi cooked *chapatis* on a flat rock. I watched her do it. Her hands skillfully shaped the cakes. She turned them on the rock and took them off just at the moment when a few black circles were forming. I felt wonderfully happy in this silence. I was grateful to Devi for having spoken of herself to me in such a direct manner, for making me touch the void. Again, this time, I found her simple, cheerful, profound. A few stones landed in the pot again. We savored the *chapatis* in silence and I retired without a word, knowing that the teaching for the day was over.

I walked slowly to the edge of the cliff. I admired the waterfall, which sparkled in the moonlight, and I went to bed, lulled by its ceaseless sound. Despite my fatigue, for more than an hour I remained still, warm enough, bathed in joy and a deep recognition. Before going to sleep, I bowed mentally to Devi. A lotus opened in my heart.

7

Devi woke me before daybreak by putting her hand on my forehead. I emerged from sleep with a mental alertness and lucidity I'd never known before. Devi carried her folded blanket under her arm. She made her way in silence toward the cliff. I got up, took my blanket, and followed her. She sat down for meditation, and just as I was about to take my place beside her, she motioned for me to sit facing her.

My meditation seemed carried by Devi's energy, which swept over me like a strong breeze and made me shiver. I felt each muscle and every nerve's desire to abandon itself totally to a sort of call from the void, so that I had to keep getting control of myself, tensing up and bracing myself to avoid being overwhelmed by what I was experiencing. Despite my resistance, I was bathed in a very strong luminosity, which lasted throughout the period of practice.

The day began, the temperature climbed slowly, and at last the first rays of sun penetrated my lined Tibetan robe to reach my skin. Devi opened her eyes wide and moved her arms. I did the same. We greeted each other at the same time.

"Did you sleep well?" Devi asked.

"Very well."

"You weren't cold?"

"No, my sleeping bag is very thick."

"And now, are you cold?"

"A little, despite the sun. I've had trouble letting go."

"That's normal. Everybody wants to let go, but how do you let go if you don't hold things, if you don't touch things in full consciousness, with a totally open heart? In Tantrism, the first thing is having the experience of touch, of profound contact with things, with the universe, without mental commotion. Everything begins there: touching the universe deeply. If you let go before touching deeply, that can bring on severe mental turmoil. Many beginning yogis make this mistake. They let go before taking hold. They lose contact with reality. The heart is never opened. They enter into a sterile void and remain imprisoned there. When you touch deeply, you no longer need to let go. That occurs naturally. The world is to be passed through in full consciousness. There is no other way, not a single detour or shortcut. When you hold something with all your consciousness, like the newborn who grabs your finger, it is enough to open your hand. Why is it that a newborn has so much strength? Because his whole being takes part in the movement that results in seizing your finger. In this instant he is so strong that you are in his power.

"Tantrism is agreeing to live out this power. The woman possesses it naturally. For her, it's easy to experience. For the man, there's only a dream of power. That's why his power is not manifested spontaneously and why it often takes a violent form. Violence is pure impotence. To be conscious of his power, a man must first come to recognize his femininity. In the same way, a woman who represses her natural power doesn't find equilibrium within herself or accept her own capacity for wonder. This is how we define the virile man in Tantrism: 'He who retains the capacity for wonder.'

"Ecstasy, the continuous experience of the divine through knowledge of our own nature, is our natural state. The infant knows this state, enjoying it from the moment of conception. It is only under pressure from the outside, education, a bad family situation, that little by little the child loses inborn capabilities—strength, capacity for wonder, absolute self-confidence, openness to the world, the free blossoming of the heart, which it learns to fold up again and then to close tight. Returning to this childlike state is the door that reopens the heart."

"Is there a difference between the natural awakening of a child and that of an adult who rediscovers this state?"

"The return to an awakened state is often made at the cost of a certain amount of suffering at the moment when the adult's armor is cracked, when the infinite slips in there. That can be an experience similar to being struck by lightning. Madness is a sort of awakening in which the lightning doesn't shatter all of the armor. The mind is halfway into the infinite and no longer recognizes the structures of the finite. Sometimes awakening is more like a glacier melting, slowly and inexorably. But often, even in this case, the consciousness goes through painful episodes. And the briefer they are, the more intense.

"When the whole suit of armor gives way to awakening in the adult, that state is both identical to the newborn's and different in the sense that it is heightened by the beauty of the journey, and it is not generally followed by regression. An adult heart that is awakened is a heart that hasn't breathed for a long time, that has retained an enormous capacity for genuine love. In seeking to let go before taking hold, one doesn't understand the profound dynamic of love, the fabulous power we all possess. We are all like bombs ready to explode with love. Even the most violent, most terrifying men and women, the ones most rejected by society because of their crimes, are not exceptions. I am here to press the detonator. What is the detonator? Sometimes, nearly nothing. Three seconds of total presence before the other will suffice. People never reach some irreversible point. Agreeing to touch the other is agreeing to make this bomb explode. It is the only solution to violence. Touch. I am going to teach you to touch. The basis of Shivaism is touching the thirty-six *tattvas,* or universal categories. It is the base on which all of Tantrism rests."

Devi let me consider what she'd said. When she paused, her whole body seemed suspended in space, in total well-being and calm openness. I sometimes had the impression that the sky and the trees listened to her, that the waterfall quieted down, that the air stopped moving. I loved the way she spoke about life, always coming back to reality and our struggle to survive, understand, love, search.

"The first five *tattvas* are
earth,
water,

air,
ether,
fire."

Devi rose, saluted space, and lay down on the ground. I imitated her, hands out in front of me, flat on the ground.

"The first *tattva* is earth. With all my body, I touch the earth. My hands touch the earth. My face touches the earth. My breasts touch the earth. My heart touches the earth. My belly and my genitals touch the earth. My thighs, my knees, and my toes touch the earth. I breathe deeply and my breath is united with the earth. The whole earth breathes. Breath is everything. I delight in the earth, its presence, its energy. The earth is real! Only your superficial contact with the earth is not real."

After a few minutes, Devi got up again and went down the narrow path that led to the river. Walking behind her, I admired the way both her feet made contact with the ground. In every movement of her body there was a grace and a presence that gave the impression of space opening to let her penetrate it.

We arrived at the basin. Devi let her clothes fall and entered the water nude. She approached me. The water covered her shoulders. She faced me.

"The second *tattva* is water. I touch the water with my whole body. The water is real. Only your superficial contact with water is not real."

She immersed herself completely. I did the same, holding my breath as long as possible. When I came up, I was astonished to see that Devi was still under water. I saw her body distorted by the water. I took another deep breath and plunged under again. I was conscious of the water going into my ears. I came up a second time and waited for Devi.

Her face emerged. She opened her eyes, and I saw in them the playfulness of a young girl. She breathed in very deeply, slowly, then breathed out. Her hair was so black it looked almost blue.

"The third *tattva* is air, which enters my lungs, then nourishes my blood and circulates throughout my entire body. The air is real. Only your superficial contact with the air is not real."

Devi got out of the water and sat down on a big round rock, face to the sun. Since she was naked, I chose another rock, some distance away, but she motioned for me to take the spot in front of her. As I sat down she said to me:

"Tantrism is one long face-to-face. Nakedness is the nakedness of the conscious in which nothing is fixed. Everything flows there like a river. The Shaktis are nude because not a single concept can find where to attach itself in their consciousness any longer. Thought itself wouldn't know how to stay put there. The phallus of Shiva is erect because it is raised to full consciousness, and in full consciousness it penetrates the universe. The vulva of Shakti is open because in full consciousness she lets the entire universe penetrate her. Shiva and Shakti are indistinguishable. They are one. They are the universe. Shiva isn't masculine. Shakti isn't feminine. At the core of their mutual penetration the supreme consciousness opens. If, in whatever circumstances, the sight of nudity awakens this revival of consciousness, then all bodies become a manifestation of the divine. Why distance yourself from the divine?

"Naked, on this rock, I am conscious of the *tattva* that is ether. It is empty space where everything manifests itself.

Even though it's impalpable, my consciousness touches it deeply. Ether is real. Only my superficial contact with ether is not real."

We waited to get dry before dressing ourselves again and climbing to Devi's hut. She rekindled the fire, boiled water and dry milk, and threw in some salt and oat flakes, which she let swell as she stirred them with a spatula. Then she made ginger tea and spread out four bowls between us. She leaned over the food and asked me to hold my hand out in front of me, open. In one swift motion, she seized an ember with her fingertips. At the moment she was going to drop it into my hand, I drew back quickly. The ember fell on the ground and crumbled.

"This is the *tattva* of fire. You didn't touch the fire. You don't have confidence."

"I have confidence in you. But with a burnt hand, how could I carry out all my tasks?"

"Sometimes my fire burns, sometimes it doesn't burn. Without total confidence there can be no spiritual transmission. You answered me, 'I have confidence in you.' But that isn't the important point. What counts is to have confidence in yourself. Absolute confidence. That's all a master looks for to kindle in a disciple. Without absolute self-confidence, there's no opening of the heart. To touch these thirty-six *tattvas* is essential. To pass through this contact opens the place where one can experience the divine. To draw back your hand is to burn yourself."

I extended my hand. I closed my eyes.

"I am ready to touch the fire."

For a very long time, nothing happened. Then I felt a sharp burning. I let out a cry and opened my eyes. Nothing except the end of Devi's ring finger was touching my hand.

She started to laugh.

"Your thinking mind touched the fire and you burned yourself. I wanted this day to be an experience of total contact with the *tattvas* for both the body and the consciousness. There is only one way to receive the transmission. When I tell you to do something, do it immediately, without the least wavering of thought. That's it. Learn. Open your heart and act. Thought stops action. It perverts it into a calculated gesture stripped of all its grace, all its efficiency. To come back to an action that went wrong makes it worse. That's only to sink deeper into the mental. Remorse paralyzes, hesitation eliminates beauty from action, thought shrinks from the world."

Devi seized my hand and, with lightening speed, flattened it against the coals. I let out a cry and instantly withdrew it. There wasn't a single mark on it or any sensation of burning. The coals, nevertheless, had been crushed under my palm. Devi looked at me with a sort of serene and mysterious half-smile that gave her face a full, radiant expression.

"Now you have touched the *tattva* of fire."

I remained silent, looking at my hand as if I expected to see blisters appear. Small stones landed in the pot. I drank some tea, then thought about this feeling of holding back, of resistance, that I had had during meditation. I spoke to her about it.

"Our strongest resistance is the resistance to ecstasy because we sense that to succumb to it we must abandon all certainty, abandon what we have put so many years into constructing. We must abandon our philosophy of life. Our beliefs, our ideas, even the concept of the void, even the concept of the absolute or of Shiva stand in the way of ecstasy. It is relatively easy to abandon fashionable ideas. It is much more difficult to give up philosophical and religious concepts. One proudly proclaims oneself an atheist, believer, Buddhist, Christian, Muslim, Hindu, tantrika. The divine can't be grasped in this manner. What's the difference between an atheist and a believer? Nothing. They are two sides of the same coin. It isn't a matter of believing or not believing. It's a matter of communicating with the nature of one's mind. It's like diving into a lake. Too often, we want to lose ourselves conceptually in the teachings as they unfold to us, and without realizing it we build a coat of armor against the divine. The most subtle teachings must be abandoned along the way. The tantrika's courage is in letting go of teachings once they've been absorbed. Even the Tantras aren't worth any more than a skin abandoned on the stones by a molting snake. When one is constantly changing, there comes a day when the consciousness rests on nothing. Then awakening occurs. Only total abandonment of the mental can open us to the divine."

"Is awakening subject to transformation?"

"All nature is subject to transformation. An awakening that isn't in accord with the deep nature of things gradually becomes diluted. One morning, you open your eyes but you're no longer awake."

"A Ch'an master speaks of the slow polishing of the awakening."

"That's it. It's not enough to find a raw nugget. It's necessary to let life run over it until the gold dazzles the entire universe."

Devi ate slowly. Each of her movements was in harmony; each mouthful seemed to bring her profound joy. This way of absorbing herself in things extended to her every activity. I had the impression that nothing was done mechanically. With her, everything was an occasion for communicating deeply, for remaining always anchored in reality. Thus, everything she did became a teaching for me. Through my association with her, I noticed those "holes" that punctuate our daily lives when we completely lose consciousness of the moment and of the divine harmony as well. It worked like real magic in Devi's least gesture, action, expression. It was as if the flow of time suddenly found itself slowed down by a dance partner from reality. Devi took up where she'd left off in her teaching.

"The so-called subtle *tattvas* are
smell,
taste,
form,
touch,
sound.

"The first is the heart of the smell. By breathing in your oatmeal gruel, you smell the odor of the oats, but the heart of the odor is not the odor. Close your eyes. Breathe in. Breathe in the world at hand—the world of fire, ashes, clothes, the hut, the forest, the water, the sky, the universe. Only then does your consciousness penetrate to the heart of smell. The heart of smell is real. Only your superficial contact with the heart of smell is not real.

"Next comes the *tattva* of taste. Take a bit of oatmeal. Savor it. Penetrate to the heart of taste. Taste the reality of this heart, which contains all the tastes of the earth. That's what must be penetrated. It's in this sense that the Tantras say one attains 'the unique savor.'

"The *tattva* of form, the heart of form, is found in the formless, which is the matrix of all the forms in the world. Like the oat flakes, which have lost their own form in the cooking, know the heart of form by following this dissolution, which takes place throughout the universe.

"You can gain access to the *tattva* of touch by touching my hand. What do you feel?"

"Your skin, your flesh, your bone . . ."

"You feel the heart of touch. Your skin and mine brush against each other. It is as if all your skin has touched mine. A shiver runs through your whole body, and you enter into the heart of touch. Through me, the universe slips under your hand. Is it possible for two skins to touch each other completely? For each millimeter of your skin to touch each millimeter of mine?"

"It's impossible."

"Then what is love?"

I remained silent, without response, and profoundly moved.

"Is it possible for each millimeter of your consciousness to touch each millimeter of the divine?"

"Yes . . ."

"Do you hear me?"

"Yes."

"Then it is the *tattva* of the heart of speech. To cross through it, you listen to the entire universe. It's in this sense that all that's heard in the universe is the mantra, AUM. All mantras are contained in the mantra AUM. Close your eyes. Listen to the mantra. . . . Only when you've heard it without a pause for three days and three nights will you be able to say it. To chant a mantra before having heard it is to arrive at death before being born."

We finished our breakfast. I felt myself entering a new universe—a universe of extreme richness. I tried to be fully attentive to all that Devi said to me. At the same time as she captivated me, I was momentarily taken by a kind of fear. What would this upheaval lead me to? How was I going to emerge from this total calling into question of my frenetic way of apprehending life? What did that enigmatic smile hide, and what would I suffer for experiencing the revolt that Devi had predicted? Many times I had the desire to take to my heels, go back down to Delhi, taste the easy pleasures, leave India for the less mystical territories of Southeast Asia. When these impulses came over me, nearly as quickly I realized that an opportunity like this—to go all the way to the end of myself—might never present itself again, and I would spend the rest of my life regretting it. This way of touching the world is marvelous, but it also contains something terrifying for a Westerner: the harrowing sense, at the beginning, of being dissolved into the objects of perception. We have reinforced the ego in such a way that it's painful to begin to feel how quickly it evaporates when we really touch the world.

"Does one practice these relationships with the *tattvas* like a sort of meditation by choosing one or another? Is that fundamental in Tantrism?"

"What's fundamental isn't to concentrate on this or that *tattva* as a particular form of meditation, but rather to realize that permanent contact with the thirty-six *tattvas* in full consciousness is the Tantric practice. Life isn't divided up like a rice field. We are subject to permanent and simultaneous contact with many *tattvas*. The being's total engagement traveling through the web of the various categories is what constitutes Tantric experience. Let's go walk in the forest and meet the other *tattvas*."

8

As Devi moved through the forest she looked to me like an image from a slow-motion film, her whole body harmoniously engaged in the walk. I tried to imitate her and realized at once how jerky my movements were. My muscles weren't accustomed to providing smooth effort, perfect balance, presence with each step, fully conscious of all the body mechanics that make walking possible, from planting one's feet on the ground, one after the other, to balancing one's arms.

"Slowness is a divine thing. We have lost the habit of it. With slow, regular, harmonious movement, the consciousness immediately finds its place. The body begins to enjoy the smallest thing. Attention is heightened. We take in the world's full freshness. We communicate. We open our senses to the plenitude. Consciousness of the thirty-six *tattvas* is an apprenticeship in completely restoring our ties to the universe, beginning with the basic elements and arriving at the divine. It's essential to feel the reality of the world in its entirety. Without that, any spiritual quest is illusory. To be entirely present to each thing that crosses our consciousness, to our most banal and repetitive experiences, is the door to awakening. Tantrism rejects nothing. All mental and bodily processes are wood, which we add to the great fire that consumes the ego and leads us straight into the absolute. This forest we're walking in—it's the absolute. There's no border between the phenomenal and the absolute. They interpenetrate each other completely. Those who don't know that look for the absolute at a great distance from the phenomenal. They impose all sorts of austerities upon themselves. They fear reality and stop playing with life, submitting to it as a kind of punishment. Their consciousness wilts like a flower cut off at its roots. In Tantrism, we throw our entire beings in, endlessly, without distinguishing between pure and impure, beauty and ugliness, good and bad. All the pairs of opposites are dissolved in the divine. The deepest urges, the most sublime capacities—no one lacks them. We begin to communicate with the divine when we totally accept the complete spectrum of our thoughts and our emotions. All beauty contains darkness. In trying to obliterate it we dry ourselves up. When one sees nothing but a singular and shared divine energy in all things, the consciousness can no longer go astray. The *sadhana* is fed by the entirety of experience, and no longer by inconsistent fantasies of purity, of spiritual realization, of power or greatness. To be nourished by purity is to be nourished by milk that has had all its nutritional qualities taken out. Those who follow this path become dry beings. Their only chance for survival is to go tyrannize another consciousness more joyous and opened to the world."

As soon as Devi evoked this sense of completeness, I realized how much I myself was obsessed with such ideas of purity and accomplishment. From the beginning of my opening up to Eastern spirituality, I had been constructing a sort of artificial ideal for myself, which could not coexist comfortably with the workings of my mind. The conflicts, the suffering I sometimes felt, the dichotomy existing between desire and realization, between sensual worldly pursuit and asceticism, had made me try to erase my dark side. Suddenly, in this close contact with Devi, I felt that old stock of repressed feelings rise up again. I felt myself discharging a great store of negativity, which the forest absorbed and which made me breath in violently, as if this internal turmoil suddenly left an empty place that allowed my lungs to find new space.

"That's good. Let all that come back to life. Breathe, participate. There's nothing that can't serve the tantrika. Breathing rediscovers the key to openness, peace, joy."

I was astonished to see the extent to which Devi's words had a physical impact on me. As soon as I came to a deep realization of what she said, my body immediately began to open, to vibrate, to release energy, to let itself be. In those moments, I often found myself wondering about the way certain Western psychoanalysts conceive of interior work. By refusing to speak to the patient and confining themselves to listening, don't they overlook a powerful tool of liberation? When the right or true word comes to strike against a paralyzing mental construction, an opening ensues—a new space where whatever suffers can finally breathe and rediscover the world. Of course, to be capable of such speech supposes that one has oneself abandoned all rigid frameworks. But without having done this, can one truly hear someone else? It seemed to me that deep listening and deep speech couldn't be disassociated, that you can't have one without the other, and that probably the great therapists are those who have access to both these inseparable tools and make use of them.

Later, Devi spoke to me about the next five *tattvas*:

the feet,

speech,

the hand,

the anus (as the excretory organ),

the genitals (as the urinary and sexual organs).

"These *tattvas* are linked to the organs of action. First of all, there are the feet, which serve to move us on the earth, to walk in full consciousness, as we are coming to do. Then there's the *tattva* of speech. I speak to you. I open your consciousness. My speech is true. The *tattva* of the hand is seen here not in the sense of touch but as the faculty for giving, seizing, moving, shaping, transforming something. I seize this branch; I can make it into a tool. I take some clay; I can make it into a pot. It's the creative capacity of the hand—that of a dancer, a musician, an artisan.

"The next *tattva* is linked to the excretory organ. It's the typical example of an activity we perform every day, which seems to us not worthy of consciousness. Tantrism tells us that to excrete in consciousness is as profound a meditation as any other. Thus, when you are going to relieve yourself, grasp this bodily movement, which takes in and rejects, which opens and closes, which lets pass through you what you have absorbed of the world.

"Next comes the *tattva* of the sex organ in its double aspect: that of urination and that of sexual use. In frenetic or compulsive sexual pursuit, the face often shows only pain, tension, constriction. When a man penetrates a woman in full consciousness, time is dilated, pleasure is extended, all the senses are opened to this experience, and suddenly the bodies truly take their place in space. Play, laughter, breathing, the shuddering of the limbs, all tend toward opening. The eyes, the intimate organs, the heart all come alive. The whole chemistry of the body is altered, the mind eases, and the brain teems. The skin softens and exhales its perfume. At this moment only, two bodies communicate deeply, and there is something of the divine in the sexual relationship. When two bodies are nude and embracing, they discover that space where they can let things be. Beginning from there, the tantrika can go much further still. But without this preliminary presence with the other, relaxed and in perfect harmony, all asceticism is bound to fail."

Devi sat on the ground. I sat beside her. She inhaled the odor of the forest. I became conscious of the space that these essences opened in me. Time became more fluid, everything taking part in our breathing. Devi took my hand, felt it, caressed it, until I began to feel overcome with heat. She spoke to me, still holding my hand in hers.

"Now we come to the five *tattvas* of perception:
the skin,
the eye,
the tongue,
the nose,
the ears.

75

"These are the *tattvas* of contact, sight, taste, smell, and hearing. These *tattvas* are subject to intense activity all day long, and we usually have a well-developed awareness of them. Nevertheless, none of them alone seems to us worthy of really practicing in full consciousness. We aren't fully conscious of our skin. We aren't fully conscious of all that our eyes see. We aren't fully conscious of the taste of the food we swallow, the lips and the limbs of those we embrace. In the world of sounds, we have only a very limited consciousness. If we close our eyes and really listen, where would consciousness stop? Until we let ourselves be carried by sounds, consciousness is closed to the infinite.

"We subject these five *tattvas* to compulsions. We lose their richness. Everything is rushed. How long since we've delighted in eating a piece of fruit? How long since kissing's made us lose our breath, feel dizzy, and blush as a wave of energy surges through our bodies? How long since our lips have traveled up and down the whole body of the one we love? How long since we've smelled the world? How long since we've sensed a being's distress or joy by the odor? How long since we've lost ourselves looking at the marvelous wings of a butterfly, at the clouds, at the stars, at the bark on a tree, or into the eyes of another human being? How long since we've understood what another human being says to us, not by the words but by the inflections of the voice, its timbre and tone?

"Without a deep connection with these things, the heart is not opened. All that we exclude from our experience because of principle, belief, fear, ideals, ignorance, or lack of attention feeds our protective systems, which are slowly transformed into prisons. The day comes when we are so well protected that others no longer even think of speaking to us, looking at us, touching us, tasting us, or listening to us. Non-communication with the *tattvas* is the material with which we construct our solitude.

"The next five *tattvas* are
the mind,
the intelligence,
the objective ego,
prakriti (linked to Shakti),
purusha (linked to Shiva).

"These are the *tattvas* of thought. The first is the matrix of thought. All thought emanates from it, without distinction. The next *tattva*, that of the intellect, or of decision and reason, guides us in our actions. The *tattva* of the objective ego is very insidious. It permeates all our actions and gives us the impression that we have accomplished this or that thing. I meditate, I am sitting, I open my eyes. It's this restrictive objectivity that brings all experience of the world back around to the ego.

"The last two *tattvas* of this group can't be separated. They form nondualistic reality. They are *prakriti*, power or nature, the goddess, united to *purusha*, the organizer, Shiva.

"*Prakriti* is the substance of the universe, its core, its fundamental power. Everything that lives is woven from this element. Whatever the shape or color, the patterns, the thickness, the size, the quality of the woven piece, it is always from the skein of *prakriti*. It's all just a web made from the primary energy of *prakriti*. The patterns evolve, change, disappear, and return in other forms, but the skein—which never stops unraveling, allowing form to enjoy its divine freedom—is constant.

"If you stay with this image of weaving, *purusha* is the weaver himself. Without the skein, he couldn't produce. The skein by itself can't take on shape. *Purusha*, then, is the principle that penetrates the material and gives it a particular form. One can't exist without the other. Whether things are clearly visible or veiled, *purusha* is the organizing principle.

"The play of *purusha* and *prakriti* is limited by the action of the next six *tattvas*, called the six cuirasses. They are

time,

space,

lack,

limited knowledge,

limited creativity,

overall illusion.

"This is an extremely important point of Shivaism, since the consciousness is founded on and set free by these cuirasses, and that's enlightenment or awakening. These cuirasses are like veils that prevent a spontaneous view of the self. Without them there would be no practice, no search. Everything would appear to us in its absolute nature.

"The first cuirass is that of being subject to the illusion that time exists and that we are bound by it. This illusion fixes us within a limited time frame. It gives us the impression that time passes. After awakening, one discovers with wonder a new terrain where nothing is subject to time. It's like waking up after a bad dream and realizing that this restriction was artificially imposed upon the consciousness. You want to laugh, to cry 'What trickery!' You want to run through towns and villages to tell everyone, but they would think you were crazy. That's the first breath of awakening.

It gives back a vitality, a color, and a clarity to everything seen outside of time.

"The second cuirass is that which makes us believe we are subject to the illusion of space and that we are located there. This illusion makes us say, 'I am in this place where my feet are planted. If I wish to be somewhere else, I will no longer be here. You have to choose to be here or there.' But really, that's not so. After awakening, we realize suddenly that we are omnipresent, and with the greatest joy, we want to proclaim this. We are everywhere. There's no point in space that is not our center. There is absolute interpenetration with all universal structures. It's like the inside of a pot. The air inside says to itself, 'The universe is tiny. I see only a small circle of sky. Around me, a wall of earth marks the boundaries of my life. What's outside?' Suddenly, Shiva comes and smashes the pot. The air that was imprisoned by restrictive thought is instantly merged with the universal air mass. That's exactly what happens at the moment of awakening, but also at death. Once the boundaries of the ego shatter, the divine returns to the divine, energy to energy, space to space, the heart to the heart. Then, anything is possible but nothing is certain. Popular teachings sometimes speak of reincarnation. The highest Tantric teachings say that fundamentally there is no birth and no death, only the illusion of being enclosed in a pot, creating the desire to be rejoined with another pot. The debate over annihilation or eternal life is something adepts transcend as soon as they recognize the nature of their own minds.

"The third cuirass is the illusion of believing that we lack something, that we are not whole. This is the illusion that pushes us to always be searching for a way, a teaching, a practice, one realization after another. It's the one that pushes us beyond the Self. It's the one that makes us unhappy, that makes us keep looking for new ways to be complete. If we lived a hundred thousand years, we would never reach the end of our quest. We would still lack something. Knowing this, the master invites the disciple to stop all external searching. No route leads to the Self. Nothing can reopen the consciousness as long as we haven't realized that we have everything within us. The true Tantric master—it's not me, nor some other; it's the Self. There's nothing to find out there. Everything divine that we look for out there is in us. To realize that is to find freedom.

"The fourth cuirass is the illusion of believing that what we can know, what we can apprehend of the absolute, is limited. We torture ourselves. We want to experience awakening. We look at the masters. We implore their blessing. We expect the gods to help us, and they look at us without understanding, because for them, we are divine, we lack nothing. So what can they do for us? We are like a maharaja who owns unlimited land and walks along the wall that surrounds his palaces, mistaking himself for a beggar. No one would give him anything to eat for fear of insulting him or being punished. We have such a thirst for knowledge that we are fooled by our power to know. It focuses on the exterior and deceives us with the illusion that we are going to find what we lack. Divine knowledge doesn't grow by accumulation. The more you try to pile up knowledge and experience, the more you paralyze your consciousness. Let's abandon this knowledge. It only inflates pride. When I say that intelligence is not the way, I don't mean to say intelligence must be rejected. I am simply saying that intelligence which accomplishes anything appears unsolicited. In tranquility it shines like a diamond. Let us return simply to the source of our consciousness and find there the treasure we sought on the outside. It's enough to sit down, to forget books and discussion, to direct our attention toward the heart. There the divine is found. There is the place of respiration where our breath mingles naturally. The infinite is no more than that harmonious breathing, free of all thought.

"The fifth cuirass is the illusion we harbor in believing our creativity is limited, sometimes even doubting that we possess the least trace of it. That's what pushes us to revere what others produce. To have beauty flow past us isn't enough. This urge, which can open us up to our unlimited creativity, is restrained by the idea that we aren't capable of such splendor. We remain without a voice, the ribcage constricted, overwhelmed by the beauty of the world. If we truly breathed, this cuirass would explode, and the object of our admiration would no longer be found in duality. The beauty of the world would then be ours. Mystical ecstasy is just this sudden explosion of the small me, which recognizes the divine Self. Everything gathered up in the consciousness is then projected into the infinite, and one can cry out in joy because in this moment all the beauty of the world becomes part of the Self.

"These five cuirasses are surrounded by a supreme cuirass, which is that of maya, illusion, in its own nature, which welds these different protective plates together and insures their artificial cohesion. We are decorated like fighting elephants, forever goaded on by their driver. We advance with all our weight to get through life, never ceasing to do battle. But one day, the battle takes a turn that leaves us covered with poisoned arrows. A young girl brings us something to drink. She speaks to us and caresses us. She dresses our wounds. She bathes us in the river, and suddenly we find our grace, our lightness, our beauty again. No one recognizes us as fighting elephants anymore. So nothing stops us from spontaneously grasping the divine in ourselves. What we don't know is that the smallest experience can be just this miraculous meeting with the small girl. So little can suffice. The scent of a flower, an open look, a breeze brushing against us—and suddenly the most solid of the cuirasses cracks, and through this gap all reality penetrates us, freeing us forever from gravity and separation."

9

I'd been living in my hut for about two weeks. Each morning, after meditation, Devi accompanied me in the perception and full consciousness of the play of the *tattvas*. Four times, the idea pot filled up with little stones, which Devi insisted I pile beside my hut and consider each morning. Sometimes she ran her hand through them and said to me, "I caress your disruptive ideas." I had the impression that the river couldn't supply me with enough stones.

One night I dreamed that I was sitting in my hut, an old man, and that in front of me was a mountain of stones symbolizing all the ideas that had cut me off from the marvelous mystical reality and blocked my view. A young girl tumbled down the slope, laughing. She approached me. I recognized Devi and woke up.

With time, the pot began to fill up less quickly. Day by day, I felt a space opening in me, and the more it opened, the more I was in a position to enjoy each *tattva* and their complex orchestration, which I spent my days and a part of my nights paying attention to. Each morning, Devi woke me a little earlier, and our meditation lasted until the moment when the sun warmed us up.

Finally the day came when she told me about the last five *tattvas*:

the consciousness taking on its true nature,

subjectivity invested with power,

the universal I,

Shakti,

Shiva.

These were not linked, like the preceding ones, to objectivity. Devi designated them as the *tattvas* linked to pure subjectivity, which culminates in absolute subjectivity.

"The first *tattva* is that of consciousness taking on its true nature, of the fragmentary and episodic realization of the Self. The tantrika is subject to ecstatic flashes, during which he perceives the universe as unreal before falling back into ordinary perception. This first state you already know. It is invaluable because it adds a real, non-theoretical picture of realization to one's practice. It's a level easily attained, once you give yourself over to continuous practice, even after only a few months. As with all progress, this first level constitutes a pitfall as well. The tantrika who isn't guided by a master can mistake these first flashes for final realization. Then he suffers from a break between the reality of the world and his ecstatic experience. He is incapable of reconciling the two. One is full of pure water; the other, full of sludge. The tantrika, at this preliminary stage, can experience a distaste for the world and decide to retire from it to preserve the purity of his mystical experience.

That's a grave obstacle to future realizations. When there's a split, there's no true spiritual life. The solitary ascetic who isn't capable of leaving his cave to exist in the world and find the same peace there lives in a state of spiritual illusion. Life is the great polisher of awakening. To flee from it for good is to flee from the highest accomplishment. It's good, on the other hand, to alternate short periods of solitude with a normal life in society. At this stage, the tantrika is still subject to duality.

"The next *tattva* is the realization of a state linked to a deeper subjectivity. The tantrika is less subject to fluctuation. He feels himself overcome by a great power. Soon he can remain in a state of ecstasy for hours without the shadow of a disruptive idea. Not a single stone goes into the pot. He feels very clearly that he flows throughout the universe. Like a breath inhaled, he lets himself go, under the impression that he enjoys the reality of the world. But his heart isn't completely opened, as he still falls back into his ordinary state in which he no longer sees the universe as an expansion of his being.

"As for the next *tattva*, which belongs to the same category of higher subjectivity, the tantrika, in the course of his ecstasies, perceives things differently still. He no longer has the impression that the universe emanates from his being, but simply that he is the whole universe, without source or flow. The source is the universe. The tantrika is the universe.

"Finally come the last two *tattvas*, which are interdependent, amorously bound to each other, and situated alone in absolute subjectivity. They correspond to the total opening of the heart. At this moment, the tantrika no longer lives as the absolute I. Duality is obliterated. This is the state of Shiva: Being in the absolute sense, symbolized by the *Aham* mantra.

"Even though we come to the end of the thirty-six *tattvas* here, there is still the Being, Parama Shiva, who escapes all qualification, all ideas. It is throughout, even in the inferior *tattvas*, and there's where the deeply human beauty and the greatness of Tantrism lies.

"Finally, not a single one of the thirty-six *tattvas* isn't saturated by the absolute. Everything is saturated with the divine; nothing can be removed from the divine. If you realize that, you grasp the true Tantric spirit."

For a few days now, after each oral teaching, Devi drew closer to me. She took my two hands in hers and, in a very soft voice, said to me:

"And now, listen with your heart. This is the most important part of the teaching, the silent teaching. What is marvelous is that the heart has *absolutely nothing to say.*"

We remained like that for about half an hour. Then, day by day, the length of this teaching became longer. The sensation that overtook me during this transmission was very special. I had the impression she let loose in me a swarm of bees, which I felt humming and infiltrating throughout as if I were a field of poppies opening their petals. I felt them gathering nectar. I was no more than pollen and honey. Very often, strong emotions were released in me during the silent teachings. Many times, I cried as if I were expelling fragments of my fundamental fear. When I had calmed down, Devi let go of my hands and we went to bathe or walk silently in the forest.

Later, seated in her hut, we ate and we drank tea, and I

asked her all sorts of questions, which she graciously answered. These were pleasant moments, a sort of game, which I found necessary and which opened large swaths of reality for me. Sometimes we had discussions while we prepared the *dal*, cutting onions, picking over the lentils, roasting the curry powder.

Often, at these times, Devi talked to me about her life and asked me about mine. The atmosphere was intimate and relaxed. Devi showed nothing of that aspect of impressive power I saw in her now and then. We were a woman and a man seated in a hut, completely occupied with the pleasure of conversation.

One day, I asked her what distinction she made between the Tantric Shivaic teaching, which sees consciousness as the receptacle of the universe, and Tantric Buddhism, which rejects consciousness as an illusory form. It was the debate between the Self and the Selfless that had mobilized great energies and had been the subject of polemics and councils, and grounds for mutual condemnation and rivalry. Devi laughed, taking on the vague and tender look she had each time she told me a story about her life.

"After leaving my master, I decided to go meditate in a cave, alone. Certain spots in the mountains, many days or even many weeks by foot from any village, have been known to ascetics for thousands of years, and often one becomes only one more occupant of a cave where dozens of sages have lived. Sometimes, one finds Buddhist sutras engraved in the stone, sometimes Sanskrit letters or mantras. The caves are often found in a place in the mountains that resembles a hive, and it happens sometimes that many dozen ascetics are living within the range of each other's voices. There you find Tibetans, Hindus, tantrikas—sometimes even Chinese and monks of the Small Vehicle with their saffron robes. I've even seen Japanese monks with their straw hats and black gowns. Sometimes, one of the hermits goes down to look for food. Sometimes they speak to each other as they draw water from the spring; they laugh and they dance, though the people in the valley can't imagine it. Sometimes a hermit dies, and they burn him or bury him or leave him to the vultures. Sometimes a hermit gets sick or is taken by what we call 'the immense fear.' All hermits know this or will know it one day. It is the ultimate crack in the Self, the doorway of the divine.

"One day, a young hermit arrived in the mountains. He must have been about twenty-five years old. He was Indian, but he had followed the teachings of a Tibetan Nyingmapa master. He had done a six-year solitary retreat, at the end of which he had decided to live as a yogi. This young hermit was not like anyone else. At first, he was taken to be mad. It happens from time to time that a hermit loses his mind and wanders about in the mountains. Sometimes he spontaneously regains his sanity, sometimes not.

"Our young Indian yogi had a hot-headed and unpredictable nature. He was noisy. He sang at the top of his voice as he explored the caves. He laughed and told funny or obscene stories. Sometimes he would shake the hermits to pull them out of *samadhi* and insult them by saying that they were lost, that their meditation was as rank as a cadaver, and that they hadn't grasped Rigpa, the pure presence. Believing him to be crazy, some laughed and others threw him out, sometimes violently. After being hit by a lot of stones, he'd calm down, but as soon as he recovered he'd start harassing us again. As for those who believed in the idea of Self, of consciousness as receptacle, he'd shout into their ears that only non-Self was supreme. As for those who clung to the idea of non-Self, he threatened to carve the consciousness to bits with a knife for them and find the Buddha there. He walked around with a large Tibetan knife, which he took out of a silver case on which the image of a dragon was engraved. Soon he was called 'Dragon.' Since he was bothering the ascetics, one of them proposed that we should meet together, and according to the ancient tradition, we should debate the question of Self and non-Self, on the condition that following the debate, Dragon would retire quietly into a cave and not trouble the ascetics anymore. Dragon accepted this proposition and saw to hawking the news of it in such a way that precisely those who weren't going to go along with the debate were his constant victims. Thus, on the chosen day, twenty-three ascetics found themselves on the knoll where the debate was to take place. According to ancient custom, the opposing sides faced each other: in one line, the partisans of Self; in the other, the partisans of non-Self. Only Dragon constantly switched sides. The debate began unenthusiastically. Then, with the skill of the arguments and the richness of the supporting citations, things warmed up, and it became a real debate. It's said that in ancient times the loser in a philosophical debate was put to death or exiled. In the scriptures, there are numerous allusions to these duels, which sometimes changed the destiny of a kingdom, as in Tibet, where

Ch'an ascetics were forced to retire after losing a debate against Indian Buddhists.*

"Dragon abused the ascetics. He jumped on their backs and cut locks of their hair. There was such fire within him; I found it magnificent. He had succeeded in making twenty-three yogis come out of their lairs. That was a feat. He didn't bully me too much. He'd come into my cave only once and, after seeing that I was a woman, had retreated.

"The debate was a wonder of humor, erudition, finesse, and skill. A few ascetics dominated. The others let them debate. Some of them had spent more than thirty years in the mountains. The clarity of their look, their beauty, their depth—it was wonderful. I savored it all. Night approached. All of a sudden, the oldest among us said that it was time to conclude. Dragon breathed his fire one last time and turned toward me. 'We have the good fortune to have a *dakini* among us. She is enjoying the debate. As for me, it

---

*The oral debate between the two schools took place in Samye, near Lhasa, around 780, and its conclusion resulted in the official ban on Ch'an, according to Tibetan sources. A Chinese layman, Wang Si, who has given a summary of the debate, defended the thesis that the Tibetan king Trisong Detsen personally preferred Ch'an, but officially adopted the Indian doctrine defended by Santarksita and Kamalasila, as conforming more to the spirit of his people, fascinated as they were with magic and occult powers.

We now know that the partisans of Ch'an, perhaps under the tacit protection of the king, would continue to practice these teachings after the Chinese masters departed, under the Tibetan names of Mahamudra and *dzogchen*. A number of texts of the teachings of great Ch'an masters exist in Tibetan translations and are there to attest, as if there were any need for it, to the depth of the mark that Ch'an has left on the highest aspects of the Nyingmapa and Kagyupa teachings.

seems that the evening is still young. I will enter into silence only if the *dakini* decides to conclude it.'

"All the hermits agreed. They turned toward me. I moved forward between the two lines. I sat down and entered into deep *samadhi*. When I opened my eyes again, it was night. All the ascetics had gone into deep meditation. Dragon was facing me. I had concluded. Only deep practice of non-duality transcends Self and non-Self. Dragon had made a wonderful incursion into our tranquility. Everyone bowed to him deeply before going back to their caves in silence. As for me, I took Dragon by the hand and performed the sexual ritual of the Great Union, or *maithuna*, with him. Then he went into a cave, and we heard from him no more."

10

Each day, Devi made me feel the reality of the world through the play of the *tattvas*. All experiences—from walking to bathing, from meditation to a meal—were occasions for remaining fully aware and present. The idea pot filled up less and less quickly. Devi's infallibility goaded me on as my mind opened up to such play and little by little lost its rigidity. Devi asked me about the teaching I'd received from Kalou Rinpoche. She wanted to know every last detail. For a whole week she interrogated me on this experience alone, especially on the deep nature of our relationship. Often, during these accounts, she let out a sort of sigh of pleasure, and she bowed, her hands in a lotus before her heart. The day when I showed her photographs of Kalou Rinpoche published in my book *Nirvana Tao*, tears came to her eyes, and she said simply:

"It's his love that made you come here. Your heart will open."

The next day, there was a fundamental change in how our days unfolded. Devi told me that I was beginning the preliminary practices for initiation and that following her instructions to the letter was of the greatest importance.

Three times we entered the river and three times we let ourselves be dried by the wind. We climbed back up the hill. Devi told me to draw some water and follow her. We forced our way into the forest. After three or four hours of walking, we stopped near a Shiva *linga* at the foot of a great tree. Near the tree was a hearth. Devi built a fire. We drank a little water before meditating and beginning the silent teaching. When we finished, the fire was out. Devi told me to undress. She rubbed my body with coals that were still warm and made me sit down facing her.

"You are now clothed in space. Your nakedness comes from stripping away all concepts. Ash is the material of the mind, calm and free of disruptive illusions. Your breathing is the divine breath. That's what I am going to leave you with here. You have nothing to do but examine the various forms which your mind is going to take on during these three days and three nights, and recognize where they come from. Fundamental fear must be perceived at the moment when we create it. Stay at the foot of this tree; conserve your water. I will come back to find you."

Devi saluted me. I bowed low. She took my clothes. I watched her disappear through the trees. Soon I no longer heard her feet. Then my panic very gradually began to rise. Even though the temperature was still mild, I began to shiver. I tried in vain to revive the fire. Not even the smallest ember remained.

By the time night fell, I had completely orchestrated my own fear, and the least little noise made me jump. Leaning against the tree trunk, watching the shapes of the trees grow dimmer in the moonless night, I devoted myself to the Shiva *linga* with exaggerated piety. The words of Ram, "This woman is very dangerous," served as my mantra.

I had the impression that all the animals of the forest came to look at this ascetic, a little pale and exuding the odor of panic through his ash garments. One night can be very long. I fabricated monsters, venomous serpents, mad ascetics springing up, one after the other, out of the forest—bears, tigers, and leopards. The dangers seemed more and more real to me. I didn't dare get up or move, close my eyes or leave them open. I imagined that Devi would never come back, that she was toying with me, and that, come morning, if I went back down to our huts I wouldn't find her there. Sometimes I thought that Devi was there, very close by, peacefully seated in meditation.

After a few hours of panic, I realized that I was hardly breathing and that, after all was said and done, Devi had left me only my nakedness, my ashes, and my breath. I tried to use it to relax my diaphragm, to produce warmth, but it was impossible for me to meditate. It seemed as though my mind had never been so exposed. Everything reverberated in it.

At one moment, I believed I heard something breathing in the night. I was paralyzed. My mind told me to get up and find a heavy piece of wood to sweep across the area in front of me, but I couldn't budge. I sniffed the night air like a small animal trying to catch the scent of a tiger. I was sure I smelled a human odor. I was about to cry out but stopped myself as soon as I realized that by doing so I risked drawing the attention of those not already there.

My teeth chattered until dawn, when, astonished at seeing nothing but trees in that first light, I fell asleep, exhausted.

When I woke up, a gentle warmth pervaded the forest. It must have been a little past noon. I got up, drank a bit of water, and took a few steps to stretch my legs, as if astonished to have survived that first night. I took the opportunity to breathe and to offer a few little mauve flowers I found in the woods to Shiva. I poked fun at myself, and without thinking too much about the night ahead, I spent the day meditating, breathing, touching the trees, and thanking them for their protection.

The panic had changed into respect but not yet into complicity, much less non-duality. I would wish so much to be a tree before the day was over!

I rubbed more ashes on my body. They formed a very soft film, allowing my skin to better withstand the cold, which had penetrated almost to my bones the night before.

As the afternoon ended I was tempted to go back down to the huts, to return to the village, then to Sonada, to Kalou Rinpoche and my little cell in the pinnacle of the temple. Surrounded by monks, keeping to the Mahakala ritual, protected by the power of my master. Then I thought about Devi again. She had warned me. There was no stopping, no turning back, no running away.

I tried to see into the future. If the test of the forest preceded the first initiation, what would the tests that followed be like? Devi had spoken to me of hatred. But for the moment, I was far from hating her. I didn't even wish for her not to be making me face my fear, face the fabrications of my own mind.

I was still pursuing these thoughts when the light began to fade. I sat down firmly at the foot of my tree and tried to elaborate a strategy for passing the second night. Breathe. Breathing seemed to me the best solution, and thanking the trees, the forest spirits, the animals, the ascetics who lived there, perhaps.

Later, before night had completely fallen, I practiced guru yoga, and, visualizing the line of transmission, I invoked the great Kagyupa sages and realized that all of them had been obliged to live in the forest and pass through their fear. I implored their aid. In that instant, it seemed that my devotion had never been so intense. I implored Devi's aid as well. When the night-blue body of Vajradhara, incarnated as Kalou Rinpoche, installed itself in my heart, I believed I felt the influx of the lineage. My breathing found its depth, warmth spread throughout my abdomen, and I rediscovered the profound sense of well-being I had known throughout the months of intense practice.

When I ended my meditation, it was night. I visualized Tilopa, Naropa, Marpa, Milarepa, the *dakinis,* Nigouma, and Sukasidha, in the company of Devi, all in a circle around me like a protective halo.

Everything would have gone well if, during the course of the night, I hadn't heard some sort of frightening grunt. Panic reclaimed me, the masters of the line went off on an expedition, Devi abandoned me, and I found myself alone again with my mind, which had now changed into a producer of horror films. Once the mind gets carried away, human, animal, and mythic monsters can spring up so easily out of nowhere!

That night, again, no one devoured me, and my devotion

extended to the trees, the stones, the roots, the mosses, and the insects. There are many to thank in a forest.

That kept me busy until evening, when I realized I hadn't even had time to be hungry.

The entire third night was taken up by an intense recognition. I was there, in the middle of this forest, which lived and let me live. Not only did it accept me, but it served as my master in showing me that I was the sole creator of my fears and my anguish.

Dawn came rapidly. All of a sudden, I saw Devi, sitting facing me, three or four meters away. She stood up and took me in her arms. In a single stroke, she gave back to me all the warmth of the world.

At that moment I felt all the gratitude that I'd experienced over the course of these three days being transferred to her. I had the impression that my whole body felt that umbilical cord she'd spoken of. It went from my belly to hers and then, like a huge red luminous serpent, passed through the bellies of everyone, the center of all things, animate or inanimate.

"Let's go down and eat some gruel," Devi said.

II

The following night, I did not sleep in my hut as I had hoped. Devi told me to rest during the afternoon. Come evening, after supper, she took me to the edge of the cliff.

"This is where you're going to meditate. Standing, your feet on the edge of this rock. Don't look at the river. Keep your eyes opened, fixed right in front of you, looking into space. When you can't stand up anymore, take the cross-legged posture and continue to meditate. When fatigue makes you slump, stretch your back and do the relaxation exercise that we call the rest of the *sarangi*. When the musician puts away his instrument, he slackens the strings one by one. Thus, imagine that your muscles are strings, that the pegs of the instrument are driven into each joint. Beginning with the feet, relax the muscles one by one, letting them bow toward the earth. Proceed in this way moving up to the knees, hips, sides, collarbone, wrists, elbows, shoulders, temples, and then to the top of the skull. When your whole body is loose, center on breathing, and relax completely. Then rest, and reverse the process, but without tightening the strings too much or tiring the instrument. After this practice, you'll have recovered all your energy."

For one second, I looked down. The cliff wasn't more than twelve meters high, but it was high enough to break bones on the rocks below. Nude and coated with ashes, I asked myself how I could maintain these three positions on the edge of the void. Devi went away, and a bit later I heard her singing, as she often did in the evening.

At first all this was not too difficult, but once night fell, the rumbling space was transformed into an abyss. I wanted to step back, to relax, to resume breathing and move on to the second position, but Devi had been very specific about the necessity of waiting as long as possible.

At this moment, the image of the body of the man pulled out of the river came to me. I didn't know to what extent Ram had been telling the truth, and I couldn't really imagine Devi capable of provoking a man's death. It had to have been an accident for which she was blamed. Perhaps it wasn't even a hermit.

The hours passed. My vigilance was wearing thin. It was extremely difficult not to move. My whole body hurt. My legs trembled, and the incessant droning of the waterfall had a hypnotic effect.

I was trying to concentrate on my breathing when, in the middle of the night, I felt a hand between my shoulder blades. I made an enormous effort not to turn around, not to let myself be thrown over the edge. One more time, my mind provided me with a series of catastrophic scenarios.

At times the hand pushed me gently forward and I resisted. At times the hand no longer touched me. Was this Devi or my imagination? If it was Devi, she knew of my fear and the existence of the body retrieved from the river.

The day, the sun, the tepid air had a calming effect. Everything seemed to be dispelled, and the three exercises flowed into each other. I discovered that Devi had left a jug of water, from which I drank with immense pleasure. I was now accustomed to days of fasting and its purifying effect on the body.

I was astonished at the extent to which the *sarangi* relaxation let me recover new energy, and the seated meditation warmed me. I felt as if I had a furnace in my abdomen. But when evening came, I found myself standing on the edge of the cliff again, and I realized how much trouble my mind had exhausting the morbid stream of images running through it.

At one point, toward the end of the second night, I was convinced that Devi was going to kill me. I raged at my Western naiveté. It all seemed absurd to me. My nerves were frayed. I wasn't far from my hut. I was tempted to run there, collect my things, and leave forever this woman whose seductive power hid a taste for manipulation—perhaps even a certain madness. I spent hours lining up end to end everything that seemed crazy and absurd to me at this moment, and I surprised myself by crying a thundering "No!" out into the night. I refused to be the plaything of a woman who, in her solitude, had lost her reason. Where would all this lead me? Wasn't there a kind of threat in her demand that I totally accept her orders? I risked great trouble! Maybe I risked even greater trouble by staying. I thought of my friend Ram, of his sincere affection and of his warnings. Well, I wouldn't have to look at Devi's wild-eyed expression, her enormous tongue, and the blood that stained her body any longer. Then, at that moment, I stretched and relaxed. I must have slept an hour or two. When I woke up, I went back to standing at the edge of the cliff.

Two nights exhausted my fantasies one by one, and by the morning of the third, I was still on the edge of the cliff, alive and standing. By this time, I'd given up fighting, and when the hand gave me a distinct shove, I gave myself up for lost, anticipating a fall, which despite everything never occurred—because, with one swift motion, Devi pulled me back.

One more time, I found myself in her arms. I had the impression that each test was helping to build an indestructible bond between us. This time, my nerves were shattered. I didn't know what I was crying about, but I was sure that the torrents of tears pouring out of me had come from a long way off.

I was entitled to an excellent meal of rice and *dal,* and to rest, which had never seemed so delicious to me. I woke several times. I opened my eyes, astonished to be there in the calm and the solitude, listening to the sounds of the forest with wonder. I was enthralled at what deep happiness the least little thing held for me, and I fell asleep again in a sort of bliss, which seemed to grow each time I reawoke. By now I had fallen into the habit of sleeping curled up like a hunting dog in the hearth pit—widened to accommodate me—naked in the soft ashes, as I had been instructed by Devi.

The following night, Devi covered herself with ashes. A crescent moon rose. Devi led me by the hand to the center of the esplanade.

"Listen to the night, the music of the stars, the songs of space."

She opened her arms and, very slowly, began to dance. She turned in circles, moving her arms like a great bird taking flight.

"Shiva is the god of the dance. Honor him until you're exhausted, and then you will fall on the ground, be whole, and transcend duality!"

Then, like her, I began turning in circles. Little by little, I felt my arms join in, tingling in space. Never had I felt such life, such a vibration rising from my legs and spreading throughout my whole body—even into my hair, which seemed to stand up as a shiver went through my scalp. There was an intense humming around my eyes, my mouth, my ears, and each millimeter of my skin danced with the night.

I felt an irresistible joy coming over me, and I broke into laughter. The more I turned, the more I laughed. I drank space, and the intoxication of being alive filled me. The steadily turning stars mirrored us like a sort of cosmic disc. Devi herself also laughed. Sometimes she approached me and brushed against me with her whole body. My penis became erect. While dancing, I felt it rooted in me as if it extended through the pubic bone. I felt like one of those ithyphallic sculptures of Shiva. We spun like naked dervishes, carrying along the earth and the sky. Sometimes Devi sang; sometimes she simply listened to the music that seemed to spring up out of the whole cosmos.

I was astonished to find that my erection elicited in me no sexual desire. It was as if the phallus rose naturally to take part in the dance. The usual mechanisms were no longer operating. I discovered, simply, the joy of a body open to space, to the night, to the divine.

For three nights we spun—playing, laughing, sometimes absorbed in the astral silence. And in the morning, we let ourselves fall on the ground in radiant exhaustion. Devi explained to me that her master had made her climb up and down mountains until this point of exhaustion, which allows us to drop and to drop hold of the root of duality.

The following night, seated in Devi's hut, I received my first initiation. Devi made a fire. I prepared two garlands of wild flowers that we exchanged. We entered into *samadhi,* and Devi performed the direct transmission, from heart to heart, which left me in a heightened, vibratory state. When she put her hand on my head, I felt a very vivid luminosity envelope me completely. She let me slowly emerge from this state, then spoke to me with such gentleness it was nearly a murmur.

"The first initiation represents the gift you make to me of the life that is beginning to be born in you. Through me, you offer to Shiva your superficial fear, vanquished over the course of these tests. You offer to Shiva your energy, symbolized by your erect phallus during the dance; you offer to Shiva the wonder that is beginning to be born in you. You offer to Shiva your laugh, your dance, your body purified by the fire of your heart. You offer to Shiva your nakedness, which symbolizes the nakedness of your heart, naked with regard to concepts, dogmas, beliefs that are the adversaries of Awakening and that no longer have a hold on you. You offer to Shiva your mind, which is beginning to quiet down, but also your raw intelligence, uncut, like a natural stone that hasn't yet passed through the hands of a jeweler. This unsolicited intelligence—it's the primal matter, vigorous, unmarked, the divine glistening through it. With culture, cutting, the intelligence may seem more brilliant, more sparkling, but it is also cut off from its original purity. Cutting, culture, makes it like other cut stones. And the intelligence, or the mind, loses its uniqueness and becomes absorbed in social games, which diminish it even as the opposite illusion is created. It's this raw material that's truly divine because it's in harmony with the universe. No one cuts the stars. No one designs the forms of the rivers; they flow by themselves. The tantrika is like a river that never stops flowing in the divine because the divine never stops flowing in it.

"In making these offerings, in receiving this initiation, you gain access to the knowledge of your own divine substance, and you open yourself to the Tantric experience of time no longer passing. Your meditation will be easier. The illusion of believing that time can be parceled out will appear to you in all its absurdity, and you will taste the nectar of undivided time.

"Initiation also involves a rupture with the myths of the specific society in which you live, establishing a profound and unconditional tie with all human beings and with all that has previously seemed inanimate to you. Initiation releases you from taboos and social, dietary, and sexual prohibitions, and more importantly, the prohibitions linked to ideas and thought. It's a liberation with regard to dogma, to belief, to doubt, and to theory. The tantrika plunges into reality with the whole bodymind. He doesn't skim; he experiments. He lives the teaching, and by his living he continues the flow of the Tantra. That's the meaning of the word *Tantra*:

continuation—continuation of the Tantric experience through the tantrika. A chain of women and men who *risk the real* and are no longer subject to the compromises social beings submit to. Initiation marks as well the secret in which the tantrika must lock himself away until the day when his heart completely opens. Only then can he identify himself as a tantrika. That's why, when you leave here, you will pretend to know nothing about Shivaic Tantrism. You won't take part in a single discussion on the subject. You won't write any books before your heart opens, keeping within you the secret of your initiations until the day when the fruit ripens. You will practice in secret, not distinguished by *rudraksa* grains, a Shivaic trident, or anything else. If, by chance, certain people talk about the Tantra, don't correct their mistakes, don't guide them, don't direct them to me or any other master. The aspiring tantrika must find his master by himself."

12

Devi waited for me in her hut. As we had done each morning since the day of initiation, we began by going down to bathe, then dried ourselves in the sun before going back up to meditate, sometimes in the forest, sometimes in Devi's hut. Then Devi gave me an in-depth explanation with commentary on each of the one hundred and twelve verses of the *Vinanabhairava Tantra,* which offer the yogi all the ways of practice and give a complete account of the teaching at the same time.

This particular morning, I felt the need for Devi's teaching on meditation. I told her this. I was seated facing her. We bowed to each other. Devi always paused before speaking. I had the impression that she situated herself comfortably in the silent space and that the words didn't come out of her mouth until I myself was also seated in that same silence.

"Meditation. It's the spontaneous experience of nonduality. In our system, there's no concentration on images, no ritual to induce the meditative state. We work with the raw consciousness without forcing it to be anything. If we make use of the mind to build something, we encumber the temple.

"I come back again to this image of the temple, of washing it down and airing it out, of the light that penetrates it, and the flight of all those voices hindering the spontaneous experience of non-duality. It's a major point, and it's the jagged rock most of those who begin spiritual quests stumble over.

"The first emptiness is easy to attain if one devotes a little consistent and regular effort to it. Clearing the temple of its little gray men—most ascetics achieve this much. Nevertheless, once the work is done, there's immense internal pressure on the adept to backslide. After years of asceticism, study, and arduous practice, those who retain the suppleness of the newborn are rare. They start to venerate an external person, external teachings, or a body of beliefs, concepts, and practices, considering them superior to all others they've known until then.

"They then take great pains to put these teachings in flower baskets and deposit them in their temples, not realizing that in this instant they've built new obstacles for their minds. No matter how great the master or the teaching, it's necessary to follow it without fixing it, without eliminating its subtle and changing character. By taking hold of something in order to systematize it, one fixes it, and in fixing it one immobilizes it. And little by little, that which we believe to be supreme is crystallized in us, grows big and heavy, and leads to our demise. Always keeping that in mind is of the greatest importance. As soon as there's a system, the Tantric spirit is lost. As soon as stockpiling begins, the Tantric spirit is lost. This awareness is what gives Tantric writings their unique fluency, like a river that can't be stopped. As soon as devotion for one's master makes us ignore the master in ourselves, we no longer take part in spirituality. As soon as we lose contact with reality in order to follow the Absolute, we lose contact with the Absolute. The entire Absolute is contained in reality. There's not a trace of it elsewhere.

"Guard the empty, open, silent temple. That's the only way to experience non-duality. As soon as any voice begins speaking inside us, we deviate from the Tantric way. True devotion, absolute love for a master, means realizing deeply that he has never said anything to us. He has only opened his heart to us so that we could see our own there. That's all. To see our hearts, our minds, to come back to the marvelous source and not lean on anything. It's a little like modeling an immense statue of Shiva out of earth. Little by little, you'd need scaffolding to reach the knees, the belly, the shoulders, the head. And when you finished, the divine would be imprisoned in a bamboo cage. As the divine breathe, a single breath of Shiva would blow the cage to bits, and the divine, liberated, would fly away with great speed. So don't do this. Don't seek the divine by constructing a cage around it. Simply breathe. Breathe deeply and no one can put you in a cage.

"All we do is make ourselves concentrate on the breath in the center of the heart. Little by little, breathing is refined and extended, and without your doing anything else at all, the chakras awaken and spring forth; the wheels begin to turn. When you inhale, the whole universe inhales with you. When you exhale, the whole universe exhales with you. To breathe is to complete an incommensurable cycle of creation, expansion, resorption, and annihilation. We are only in the exhalation phase of the universe, everything moving away at an amazing speed. One day, the universe will be in its inhalation phase and everything will draw close at the same speed. Thus, a single breath of yours accompanies the creation of the world and its resorption. When awakening occurs, one lives this explosion, which projects all the residues of the consciousness out toward infinity. But one also lives the complementary movement of resorption because it is the same image of life. Many adepts deny this phase. They don't perceive that in essence it is its opposite as well. When there's no more movement, there's no more life.

"The mind always wants to cling to concepts. From childhood it is trained to devour concepts. It is never satisfied. It always wants more of them, like a wandering ogre. In general, one spends the first part of life searching, and the rest, dying spiritually. The fatal moment when everything is reversed is the moment we fossilize our knowledge into belief. It's all the more pernicious because it's precisely at the moment we begin our descent that we have the reassuring impression of taking a big step toward consciousness.

"Very few are capable of the second temple cleaning. To empty it of all concepts, beliefs, dogma, of all ideas of the divine—that's the Great Yoga. As soon as it's accomplished, one discovers the freedom to which all Tantrism leads. That's why it's so difficult to become a tantrika and to keep your hands in the earth without ever beginning to make a model of the divine out of it. But that's how to situate yourself at the center of Self and to gain access to the heart, to the incomparable void."

Later, I asked her for a teaching on the chakras.

"*Chakra* means wheel. It's like a potter's wheel. If you push on the pedal, the wheel goes, if you don't push on the pedal, it doesn't move. In other words, we don't have chakras as long as we don't make them turn."

"In the West, we worry about our chakras, like our hearts or our lungs."

"Really? And where do you locate this subtle body?"

"Around the Self, above the Self, on some other plane. There are many theories."

"Nothing is elsewhere. Everything is here. Practice gives birth to the subtle body. Practice gives birth to the chakras. To be born, they must spin. Just as there's no infant without sperm and egg, there are no chakras without meditation and non-duality."

"On which of the chakras does one begin concentrating?"

"In our line, we don't concentrate on any chakra other than the heart. Otherwise, you risk a wild outbreak of the kundalini, which can bring on anguish, depression, or madness. We concentrate only on the breath passing into the heart. That's what everything depends upon. When the heart is radiant, empty, and peaceful, the breath rises and makes the other chakras turn. Then alone can the kundalini be released, because the passageway is not obstructed. My master, when he watched the great efforts I made to always meditate more, used to smile and say to me, 'Relax, Devi. One of the great secrets is that everything is self-made.'

"That conflicted with my determination, my vital desire to progress, to become an accomplished yogini. It would take me years to realize and accept this profound teaching. The more stages and steps there are, the more artificial the teaching is. Everything in the world becomes more and more complex, but in Tantrism it's the reverse. We move toward supreme simplicity. You look at a potential disciple. You see what his gifts and possibilities are. Then you simply keep him from applying himself too fanatically. He must be allowed to breathe, to play with time's unreality, to open naturally to the understanding that our method is extremely simple. The ancients took care to strip it of all useless ornaments. That's why not a single master adds anything whatsoever. As soon as one traces a route and sets out on it, with each step that route is lengthened by a step. In returning to one's own fundamentally pure and perfect dwelling place, one is opened to the absolute. The teaching is perfect in its simplicity. To refine or modify it is to weaken it. Any adept knows too much already. You know too much already. You're here to forget it! It's simply a matter of letting oneself be, in total freedom, until the moment when the consciousness is dissolved into the divine, just as if it were responding to a passionate kiss."

"How do you breathe during meditation?"

"Naturally. Slowly. Through the nose if your thoughts are peaceful, through the mouth if they are agitated. By letting the belly out completely while inhaling, and retracting it without force while exhaling. The diaphragm supple as a jellyfish; the anus relaxed; the throat relaxed; the brain relaxed; the cranial bones like another diaphragm; the shoulders, the arms, and the hands relaxed. The point of the tongue on the palate, against the upper teeth. The spinal column very straight, the vertebrae stacked up like little round cushions full of sand. The eyes slightly opened, fixed before you on the ground, or completely opened and fixed on infinity, right in front of you. Then, without forcing it, you extend the breath, you let it become subtle, and then you notice a pause between the exhalation and the inhalation, and you realize that the divine is in this interstitial void. Then, you practice circular respiration born of *hamsa*."

"At the beginning, when one first starts to meditate, isn't it easier to have an object to concentrate on?"

"You can concentrate on a little pebble or some other object, but you have to be careful not to do this for too long or it will become fossilized in the mind. When you meditate with some sort of crutch, you must alternate your concentration with mind relaxation like a series of waves. You must let the concentration breathe, or you wear yourself out for nothing."

"How should one consider the intrusions of thought that come to interfere with one's absorption?"

"You have to stop believing that these distracted states are at odds with profound absorption. They are a kind of energy to be grounded in the absorption. As soon as you stop considering them an obstacle, you witness a wonderful transformation in which the agitation begins to nourish the calm. There is no antagonism in non-duality. All efforts to reduce turbulence or make it disappear only reinforce it. The clouds are part of the beauty of the sky. The shooting stars are an integral part of the night. The night doesn't say to itself, 'Here comes a shooting star to interrupt my peace!' So be like the sky, and your mind will integrate all states."

"And when one leaves meditation, how does one move in the outside world?"

"It is necessary to really grasp that you don't sit down to avoid or achieve some exterior thing. You don't meditate to experiment with altered states of consciousness or whatever else. You meditate only to perceive by yourself that everything is within us, every atom of the universe, and that we already possess everything we would wish to find outside of ourselves. To meditate is to be one hundred percent in reality. And if you are in reality, what would you be leaving by entering the outside world?

"To meditate in solitude or walk amid the hustle-bustle of a polluted city is fundamentally the same thing. Only when we have realized that do we really begin to meditate. In meditating, we run after nothing; we aren't looking for any state, any ecstasy other than being totally within reality. Those who pretend to reach higher states of consciousness through meditation are only taking *bhang*.* Beginning from the moment when we are the entire universe, how could we be lifted toward anything? It's enough to open your eyes. It's all there. When we meditate in this way, seated, standing, or lying down, we overflow with the divine and the divine overflows into us."

"What is the importance of spontaneity in the life of the tantrika?"

"That's a very important question because it leaves room for many mistaken ideas concerning spontaneity. To be spontaneous is to be divine. That goes beyond all notions of the ego, of separation. An action dictated by the ego can

*Indian cannabis-based hallucinatory drink.

never have the grace of true spontaneity. The *sahajiya,* the spontaneous being, exercises a sacred freedom that cannot be confused with impulsiveness not yet permeated by full consciousness. It often happens that young adepts allow themselves impulsive, chaotic acts under the pretext of sacred liberty.

"Any act that isn't inscribed in the cosmic harmony is only an impulsive movement, a spasm of the ego. Certain Tantric masters say that it's necessary to pass through impulsiveness to exhaust it and to be able to attain spontaneity. They simply see to it that this free impulsiveness doesn't undermine the life. Social beings have been subjected to so many hazings, so many bans. They have left behind them so many half-achieved, inharmonious acts that impulsiveness can be a kind of detoxicant for the consciousness. My master often used these exhaustion techniques to bring his disciples into contact with the empty moment when nothing remains. One day, a scholar, a *pandit*, came to find him. Instead of talking to him about the void, about letting go of the mental, my master set about arguing with him for two days and a night. He didn't allow him any breaks, only enough time to drink a cup of tea or eat a *poori*, and even during these times he bombarded him with arguments and questions, contradicting all his certainties. The evening of the second day, the *pandit* stopped, exhausted. He experienced a few seconds of emptiness. The next day, teaching began. Three weeks of silence, closed in a dark room. My master had a wonderful capacity to adapt himself to each individual. He never gave the same teaching twice. I have seen him fill up an epicure with delicacies and talk with him about the culinary arts to exhaustion. He did the same thing with a man obsessed with sex who came to him with the single hope of discovering new pleasures and gaining mastery over breathing and orgasm so he could satisfy all his mistresses. Day and night, adepts passed through his room, one after the other. The man went beyond his wildest dreams and then regained equilibrium by passing through the void, the empty moment."

"Your master shrank from nothing."

"No. He had the art of pushing all situations to that point where action is resolved into peace and quiet. One day he found himself facing a disciple with a very violent nature, who, when he was given the freedom to do what he wanted, jumped upon my master as if to kill him. My master grabbed a log and knocked him out. When he came to, the disciple expressed his disappointment, which we shared. We didn't think our master ought to have resorted to violence. He answered simply, 'I have many memories, and I only did that to remind me of my own impulsiveness. It was a completely spontaneous act.' The lesson was very effective. That disciple has become one of the most deeply spontaneous adepts of our group."

"What's the connection between the unconscious and the spontaneous?"

"What you call the unconscious, we call the deeply conscious, and it is the field we never stop sowing with all our unspontaneous acts. When we meditate, we let the jar that holds the consciousness rest, the unconscious or the deeply conscious included. When we live impulsively, this jar is forever being shaken up and made cloudy. The sludge and the water are so completely mixed up that any examination of the contents is impossible. When we meditate, we stop agitating the jar and set it down before us. Little by little, the water clears, and the deep seeds float to the surface. That's what sometimes makes the meditation process so painful. It reveals the seeds that we don't want to see in ourselves, or that we didn't suspect existed. Little by little, the contents of the innermost depths of the consciousness appear on the conscious surface and are purged. By meditating, we accept the opening of the jar and the purging of all that appears on the surface of the water. If at the same time we attain spontaneity, we no longer sow the deeply conscious field, and little by little the cycle is broken.

"As a result, the contents of dreams change. Adepts achieve full consciousness and divine spontaneity even in their dreams, which are no less one with the absolute. As long as duality remains on the level of dreams, awakening isn't complete. The ascetic who seems to have achieved Selfhood, but who is secretly tormented by his dreams, lives a lie. Everything in the Tantric *sadhanas* aimed at satisfying the senses comes from a profound understanding of human nature. Human nature can never be really opened to ecstasy until everything that was imagined, but not experienced as a result of morality or social repression, can finally be enacted with divine spontaneity. In this way, the Tantric adept doesn't leave a single hidden residue, a single unsatisfied desire, a single dream remaining within, that can't be discharged through the *sadhanas*. That's a major point of the Tantric quest. All repression that isn't flushed out or satisfied produces beings tormented by the spirit. They will never achieve divine spontaneity. This is one of the reasons why Tantrism is sometimes misunderstood by Hindus and probably also by Westerners who see an opportunity for impulsive debauchery where the divine exercise of spontaneity and the radical elimination of unsatisfied desires intersect."

"Is that why you told me there were no sexual rites in Tantrism?"

"Any sexuality that doesn't grow out of divine love is only a sham you might abandon yourself to, which you can't call Tantrism. Any experience linked to the ego, desire, or possession has nothing to do with Tantrism. To become a tantrika you must have the soul of a hero. Under no circumstances can someone ruled by passions or victimized by an egotistical, manipulative sexuality complicated by power or repression advance successfully along the way. When Shiva penetrates Shakti, it's a complete act, a sacred act. Without the triple mastery of the breath, the mental component, and the sperm, it's the very same act that has chained beings to ignorance since time began. They come together without realizing that everything within is divine, as if suffering in the form of a penis were penetrating suffering in the form of a vulva. Despite that, and even carried out within the suffering ego, the sexual act contains the whole of divinity, though it's not apparent to most, for whom sexuality is so troubled. But it's really so simple! It's only our fragmented and dualistic minds, our knowledge turned outward, our ideals and morals that hide from us the knowledge that we are gods!"

13

Devi woke me before dawn. She looked happy, like an adolescent preparing for an important event.

"Let's go down to the river and bathe. We're going to town!"

"To town?"

"Yes, there are things to buy. We're out of supplies."

I was amused at the prospect of making my way through the noisy town with Devi. As soon as we returned from bathing we did a short meditation, and then headed down toward the village to the bus stop.

A few hours later we were immersed in the hubbub, the pollution, the colors, the hectic town life. Only five weeks before, I'd built my hut, and already the shock of town was intense and astonishing to me.

Seated in a rickshaw, we watched with wonder. Devi was wearing the white shawl I'd given her. We stopped at a dairy shop to eat a dish of yogurt, thick and sweet-tasting as cream. Then Devi asked the rickshaw wallah to head toward the suburbs, where there was a sort of shanty town.

As we went from the heart of the town to the outskirts, the bright colors of the saris, the facial expressions, and the looks gradually changed. Everything seemed more monochromatic, more sad. Only the children were still unmarked by misery. Devi observed me. All of a sudden, when we arrived at the outer fringes of the town, something changed again. That wasn't immediately apparent to me. At first, I noticed the sores on the faces, hands, and feet, the arms and legs bandaged in rags. Then I saw one face after another in which everything seemed to be decomposing. Only then did I realized we were among lepers.

The shock was violent; the contrast between the life I knew and the depths of human misery, piercing. I was acclimated enough to India to know how common this type of experience was and how difficult it was to oscillate between India's splendor and its brutally exposed suffering. The further in we went, the more looks turned toward us. I went through a series of emotions hard to identify: fear, disgust, followed by shame at falling prey to these feelings, at seeing how little all my practice had changed this duality in me. I had trouble accepting it, all the more so because Devi's presence made me feel everything so violently. My feelings alternated between pity and repulsion, disorientation and coldheartedness. It was as if I were paralyzed by the fact that each of these emotions would be perfectly transparent to the clear-sighted Devi. I believed I could get out of it by speaking.

"It's terrible," I said.

Immediately I saw Devi's look turn dark. She asked the rickshaw wallah to stop. The lepers approached us, moaning and extending their hands. They touched us, begged us for alms.

"'It's terrible' doesn't mean anything. It's an escape. You are paralyzed by fear and disgust. A tantrika confronts his fear and disgust. Get down, move among them, take them in your arms, open your heart. I will come back to find you tomorrow."

I got down, my legs hardly able to support me. I watched the rickshaw drive away. An enormous wave of nausea came over me. Retching, I fell to my knees to vomit. One hand, then another came to rest on my shoulder. Someone brought me water. I was the one who needed help. I took in the general mood. We were human beings. The umbilical cord Devi had told me about was palpable. All of a sudden the cliché according to which I was there to give something to the lepers shattered into bits. Everything was reversed.

I stood up and immediately experienced a change in perspective. Everything had happened so quickly, the transition from repulsion to acceptance was so sudden, that a great emptiness opened within me. All was calm. I had needed them and they had brought me aid. A very strong emotion came over me. I could rise and take these men and women into my arms, without disgust, recognizing what they had done to touch my entire being, what they had helped me to overcome. It would be necessary for me to surmount a series of tests in the next few hours: to drink and eat with them, to visit the bedridden. The lepers thought that I was a doctor.

Panic rose again somewhat when night fell and made it necessary for me to accept a mat under a sheet-metal and cardboard shelter. I didn't sleep. I watched the large, inquisitive rats. The stench made breathing difficult.

During those still hours, people coughed or moaned. The atmosphere was simultaneously serene and apocalyptic. Weight, gravity, infinite suffering could be read in each look, but at the same time there was levity and a sort of luminous resignation, which was the most moving thing of all.

I had wanted to leave my clothes behind and flee. The next moment, I was bursting with gratitude for those who had let me touch the depths of my fear, repulsion, and anguish. I had the impression that I'd reached whatever it is at our base that separates us from others, whether they are healthy or sick. It is a very hard pit that we protect and preserve, often by our charitable acts themselves. We are ready to give anything so that we don't have to give ourselves.

In the morning, I shared a plate of rice with the family that had welcomed me. I drank from their water. I felt happy but also very fragile, as though my well-being, my health, were an extremely delicate veil that was longer sufficient to make me different from those around me. I thought of what Devi had said about the ascetics who weren't capable of going down into town, into life; the state they enjoyed had become a way to separate themselves from the world.

When I heard the rickshaw bell, my heart leaped. I remembered that my first thought had been "How am I going to survive until tomorrow?"

I was there, alive, and free of my disgust, my fear, my repulsion, my impulse to flee, and my false pity. In one night, I had learned more about my relationship to others than in seven years of practice. Reality had seen to opening up deep communication and getting me in tune with the other. I vaguely understood that disease was only a superficial facade for this initiation. The real base was simply the other, which presents itself when the ego implodes. It wasn't a matter of giving a little or a lot, of giving anything at all. It was simply a matter of giving oneself. It's this gift that the ego refuses most stubbornly to make.

I bowed deeply before those who had taught me so much. They returned my salute, and I climbed back up into the rickshaw. In the afternoon, I bought one hundred kilos of rice and took it to them. Now that I had given myself and received so much in return, I could give something material. The gesture was no longer an evasion. It was simple, profound, and real. Since that day, I have never again felt repugnance for a human being, no matter what his or her state of physical decay.

Devi didn't say a word about this experience she'd imposed on me. That I'd passed the test led to no acknowledgment on her part. This was nothing more than a normal experience of the inflated ego coming face to face with reality.

Devi had regained her good humor. She stopped at a bazaar to look for a toy seller. She showed me some little painted metal boats that moved when a candle heating a water pipe produced steam to propel them. She bought five colored pinwheels. I bought pants and a tunic of light cotton and rolled my soiled clothes in a newspaper. We bought a few bags of grain and lentils and finished our shopping in a back courtyard, where Devi asked for a bottle of *bhang*, a milky greenish liquor. I was astonished by this purchase, but she told me that we needed it for a ritual we would be practicing soon. I asked her a few more questions on the subject, but she didn't answer me. I knew that Tantric ascetics sometimes use *bhang* in the three-M ritual aimed at destroying the dietary, sexual, and inhibitory prohibitions of the consciousness. The three M's correspond to three *tattvas* of the first group:

Ether corresponds to sexual union *(maithuna)*.

Air corresponds to the use of alcohol or narcotics *(madya)*.

Fire corresponds to meat *(mamsa)*.

Loaded down, we climbed to our hermitage, and Devi began to detach the pinwheels from their wooden supports to fix them one on top of the other along the length of a pole, which she then planted in front of the hut. The air set them spinning. Devi watched with wonder. We coated ourselves with cold ashes. Standing, and assisted by the pinwheels, Devi instructed me on the five chakras, touching the points on my body to which they corresponded.

"*Muladhara* is the chakra of the foundation, of earth. It is located here, between the anus and the perineum. It is the place of pleasure, of contact with the earth, but it is also where the ego and its associated obstacles are rooted.

"*Nabhi* is the center of the navel. It corresponds to fire and is linked to emotions, feelings, egotistical love, fear, violence, and pride.

"*Hrdaya* is the center of the heart. It is the seat of the breath, the Self, absolute love. It's the place where discriminating thought is extinguished to make room for the divine. *Hrdaya* is at the center of the body. Two chakras above, two chakras below. It is the center of anxiety as well.

"*Kantha* is the center of the throat. It is linked to the truth, to the profound word, and to sacred song but also to lying and to false situations.

"Last comes the *bhrumadhya* chakra, between the eyebrows. Linked to the sun and the moon, this chakra projects energy toward the opening of the fontanel, or the *brahmarandhra*, to reach Shiva in *dvadasanta*, in the space above the skull.

"During practice, imagine that the lowest chakra and the highest chakra are connected by a tube of light in which an infinite number of wheels are put into motion. One thus retains the idea of ascending energy and avoids being blocked by a visual image or concept of localized chakras. The chakras are often lived by yogis as stages and thus as blocks. If they are imagined as a continuous tube, nothing conceptual can come to block or limit the energy of the *kundalini*."

Later, we danced for part of the night. There was a moment when our turning became regular, almost slow motion, and the trees and sky became two masses finding equilibrium, dark and blue discs becoming blurred and rectilinear as in an infinitely blown-up photograph.

That night my first initiation into sexual practice took place. It was the beginning of a course that slowly cut the body off from its habits, actively demonstrating how our habitual sensuality is arbitrary and limited. These strange practices led, step by step, to a complete deprogramming of the automatic sexual responses and finally allowed for the practice of the Great Union.

While we danced, Devi went to find a bottle of oil we'd bought at the market, and, all the time dancing behind me, she massaged my spinal column from the nape of the neck

124

to the coccyx. Our dance became extremely slow. Devi told me to concentrate on the moon while her fingers came and went over my backbone. I had the impression that her movements melted my vertebrae, one by one, and gave them the suppleness of a single stalk that supported my body.

Devi sang, her voice never climbing above the lowest registers, and I had the sensation that she was singing in the flexible cord of my back. I started shivering intensely, vibrating like a violin string, my gaze lost in the pale crescent of the rising moon. Little by little, these sensations would build and pass from the coccyx to my penis, which seemed a natural extension of my backbone. As during the first time, my penis became erect, arcing toward the moon, but this time my whole being shuddered, and I felt a sort of resonant humming that began in my spinal column and spread throughout.

Devi continued to massage me, never going below the coccyx. She stopped singing and began to breathe more and more deeply. I breathed with her, still fixed on the moon, feeling the sexual excitement mount in me as if it crossed through the elements, entered through the soles of my feet, and traveled throughout my entire body.

The waves of orgasm swelled very gradually, accompanied by the breathing, and three or four times I projected my sperm out into the night. Devi held me against her. I felt her warm body imprinted against my thighs, my back, my neck. I had climaxed without any direct sexual stimulation, and Devi took me in her arms, our bodies moving imperceptibly, united in the night.

"Offer these lunar pearls to Bhairavi, the Great Shakti," murmured Devi.

The next day, Devi told me that three days of fasting and solitude in the forest were going to lead me to the fundamental experience of meeting Kali. I entered the forest naked with my water jug and forced my way alone to the place where I had passed my first test. I had no difficulty sleeping. The following morning, I entered into a deep *samadhi*, free of blinking, swallowing, and mental digressions or distractions. A deep devotion to Devi filled my heart, and my peaceful breathing came to rest and be reborn there with calm and regularity.

One's perception of time is strange in the forest without means of measuring it. Everything begins to expand. Being is dilated and, little by little, loses its relationship to duration, although the shade from the trees shifts and the descending light is accompanied by a coolness that seems to slip from between the length of the trunks.

I experienced a sense of opening that seemed to have no end. I considered my former fears with an amused smile. I mistakenly believed myself free of the panic that sweeps through all reality.

The many noises riddling the night no longer disconcerted me. I relished this solitude, never imagining that it was a prelude to the most terrifying experience of my life.

14

Devi opened the bottle of *bhang* and told me to drink it. We were seated facing each other. Without a second thought, I drank the *bhang*. I placed the empty bottle near the fire and looked at Devi. She smiled at me and then immediately entered into *samadhi*. I joined her, her presence making the passage extremely rapid. A blink of the eyelids, a single breath, a perfectly relaxed posture, and my whole being was floating on an ocean of milk.

Thanks to Devi, I had succeeded in perceiving how natural and near ecstasy is to us. The conceptual barrier through which we enter it is fragile. Our resistance to ecstasy is no thicker than a paper wall. There comes a moment in meditation when one notices a tension manifested as a trembling, which one hesitates to go beyond because it's the last holdout of one's fragmented bodily consciousness. The day when one takes this minuscule step, the body abandons itself completely, and one passes over to the other side of this vibration to enter into an infinite landscape, that of empty consciousness.

Then, in this void, began the dance with Devi, very slow at first, then faster and faster, under the stars and the moon, in the echoing roar of the waterfall. Our ash-covered bodies played with the universe. Little by little, the trees, the earth, each particle of dust entered into this unlimited movement.

I felt the trance slowly coming over me. In the moonlight, the ashen body of Devi was transformed into that of Kali, the black goddess who embodies liberating energy in its most terrifying aspect but who destroys illusions and opens the door to the absolute Self under this aspect as well. This power transcends time. She pulled me into the infinite, made me feel the fragility of my temporal armor. I had the impression of emerging from it, as out of a chrysalis, into blinding clarity. I was at once helped and hindered, freed and wounded, by my resistance to the goddess. Her eyes rolled; her terrifying look paralyzed and captivated me at the same time. Her destructive power seized hold of my understanding and my grounding. The more I resisted, the more devastating her strength seemed. Everything with a name, all forms, disintegrated when they came into contact with her black flesh. The chain of decapitated heads that she wore rattled and hissed, the faces twisted with pain letting out sighs, groans, and blood, which ran down her supple, structureless body. I felt her to be as powerful as the cosmic core, black as coal, unbelievably massive and compact, and defiant of illusory time.

Kali turned toward me, waving her four arms, her wild hair flying out in space, her bloodshot eyes holding me powerless in their terrifying light. Her huge red tongue lolled, trembling, from her mouth. She brandished a sacrificial sword and made *mudras* with her two right hands. A kind of symphony of groans and moans took possession of me, and the fifty heads in her macabre necklace turned like a lasso, the faces growing and shrinking so violently that I lost all sense of my size in relation to the surrounding space.

Little by little, Kali began to make menacing gestures. Her free hand took hold of my hair as the sword swung around in space to find the ideal angle for my decapitation. My bellowing supplanted that of the already cut-off heads. Kali pinned me by the hair. I saw the sword fall, and I felt it cut through nerves and tendons, arteries and muscles, trachea and vocal cords with indescribable slowness and precision. Finally my head was detached from my body, my neck retracted, and my thoughts emptied into space. Kali, dancing, made my heavy head turn. Only my eyes were still functioning, and I saw clearly dark space, the moon, and the blood on Kali's black skin.

The revolving motion increased. She let me go, and I was projected into the distance like a cannonball of brains and bones. My head rolled; I felt the ground; I saw the dust and sky. Far off, my pale and headless body staggered about and finally collapsed. Kali stamped on it, dancing on its limp surface. Then she stood still, and I felt the whole weight of her body sinking into mine. The sacrificial blood splattered all over me, and my far-off head shrank. Victorious and dominating, Kali fed on my darkness. With one terrible look, her tongue quivering, she absorbed it in the black depths of the night.

The more I was emptied of my shadow, the greater was my sensation of having touched the very bottom of metaphysical fear. The mystical devouring of which I'd been the sacrificial subject gradually returned me to a new body streaked with light as if it were larded with an ever-increasing ecstasy. My light and empty head flew up to rejoin my body. Bit by bit, the image of Kali dissolved. She lost her terrifying attributes. And as dawn took the sky I recognized Devi, bending over me, her look overflowing with light. She gently caressed my forehead as one would an infant's who was waking from a nightmare. I resumed my place in my body, and there was no more blood or terror.

I had come through the great metaphysical fear. I recognized the sound of the waterfall, the edge of the forest, the forms of the mountains and hills bathed in the twilight glow of innumerable reds, the Tantric color *par excellence*. There are often striking sunrises and sunsets in the Himalayas. The clear air and rapid cloud movement, the changes in the spectacular sky never ceased to fascinate me. From gold to lava, then to blood-red—all the colors crossed the sky.

Devi accompanied me to my hut and wrapped me in a blanket. I laid my head on her crossed legs, nestling against her crotch, where I listened to my heart beating and fell asleep.

It was in a dream that I received the next initiation. I was in my hut. Devi sat facing me and told me that initiation through dreams possessed strong power and thus it was sometimes used in her tradition. Initiation in the form of a dream had the particular ability to gather all the levels of consciousness onto the same plane, and this was precisely the reason for its great reputation among yogis, not only in Shivaic Tantrism but in Tibetan Tantrism as well.

The dream transmission was a symbolic one in which the master hardly spoke. I watched Devi's lips move and heard:

"The severed head, the offering of your intelligence.

The fusion of colors and opposites in the black skin.

The nakedness, the illusions set free.

The severed heads, its central omnipresent power.

The sacrifice, the birth of the empty fetus.

The trampling of the corpse, the rupture of bonds.

The rebirth, the absolute freedom."

The days that followed passed peacefully. Devi didn't give me a single order.

"Do whatever you like," she told me, with that playful young girl's smile of hers.

Then I discovered the phenomenal freedom of waiting for nothing, pursuing nothing, anticipating nothing, making no plans. I took unimaginable pleasure in letting myself be. We bathed, we strolled through the woods at night like two ash shadows, we ate, we danced, and the moon moved toward its fullness.

15

One evening, Devi had me lie down on her blanket. She began singing while her hands, which she'd passed through the warm ashes, traveled up and down my body. She taught me the twenty-one secret energy points that are stimulated in massages and union rituals. I closed my eyes and released myself to her caresses, which continued for hours. I felt each fiber of my body awaken to pleasure. The energy bonds grew little by little, and every part of me opened to all the others in a magical humming. My cells glided along in the stream of her voice, which played a part in my ecstasy. I began to vibrate like the string of a *sarangi* against the bow, and I emitted my own music. I felt the deep muscles of my abdomen relax and my legs shake. The strangest thing was that I had several orgasms followed by ejaculation, even though I had no erection.

I floated in sleep watching the beautiful face of Devi. I had experienced orgasm without direct sexual contact, orgasm without erection, and I suspected that I still had other discoveries to make.

A few days of leisure intervened between each of the diverse experiences that Devi put me through. They introduced me to a fundamentally different relationship not only with my body but with desire and possession of the other as well. Although Devi made me go through intense erotic emotions, never did it occur to me to embrace her, take a turn at caressing her, or make love to her. I was completely absorbed in discovering another way of envisioning my relationship to the female, to the divine, and to sexuality.

The next stage of my initiation into Tantric sexuality was even more strange. That night, near a good fire, Devi rubbed my body with oil and massaged me for a long time, sometimes brushing against my penis so that it became erect. Then, making me feel with her index finger the extremities of my deep stomach muscles, she asked me to breathe deeply enough to feel the air going from these points, near the pubic bone, to two points situated under the clavicle. That required extremely deep breathing, long and gradual, the effect of which was to make my penis go limp, its sexual charge dispersed throughout the entire body by the depths of my exhalations.

As soon as I stopped breathing this way, my penis grew hard again and was recharged with a very localized excitation. After an infinite succession of these respiratory waves, I had the sensation of having a kind of dam around my penis, its floodgates opening as I wished, thus letting the waves of excitement spread into every hidden recess of my body.

For the moment, only the current of erotic excitement ebbed and flowed, but over the course of the nights that followed, I learned how the paroxysms of ejaculation could also be controlled by deep breathing, ebbing and flowing without the least frustration, since orgasm was really taking place but was not accompanied by ejaculation.

It must have taken about ten days for this stage to become a reflex in me. Each evening, Devi introduced me to the most subtle erotic sensations; then, using her hands or breasts or mouth, she slowly brought me to orgasm. At the moment of ejaculation, using her index and ring fingers, she pressed hard against a point situated between my anus and perineum or on another point three finger-widths above the right nipple. I then had a violent orgasm without the slightest trace of ejaculation.

Then, slowly, she brought me right back to what had seemed an insurmountable threshold, making me discover pleasures more and more intense, eliciting a series of orgasms during which I lost not a single drop of sperm.

Over the course of the nights that followed, Devi taught me to achieve the same results myself without the finger pressure, simply by controlling my breathing and relaxing my deep stomach muscles. At first, there were a few accidents to which she responded with laughter. The reflex wasn't established for some days, but soon I succeeded in controlling ejaculation during totally free orgasms by myself. And believe me, this had nothing in common with the dreary *coitus reservatus*, contrary to what certain Tantric scholars claim.

In the beginning, Devi paused briefly at the moment of climax; then, little by little, she continued her stimulation, increasing the pressures of her tongue and her mouth as if to evoke my orgasm despite my deep breathing. Many times, she succeeded in making me come, which amused her no end.

It was only after a good month of these very Indian games that I achieved the mastery necessary to practice the Great Union.

"All this apprenticeship is aimed at transforming the man's ordinary and mediocre climax into a climax of slow and constantly increasing waves, which makes him capable of experiencing the pleasure of the woman and honoring the goddess as he should. The normal male orgasm is an act of violence against the woman. It's an expression of male impotence, using this brief pleasure like a knife to take a stab at all that's hidden deep within her infinitely capable body. When the tantrika discovers that his pleasure is no longer bound up with coming as quickly as possible, too quickly to satisfy a woman, he discovers all the richness of his feminine side. And discovering that, he rises to the power of the woman and the part. Even the most subtle lovers, if they don't know the secrets of Tantric *sadhana*, are privy to only the smallest part of the pleasure they could give. The male body is numbed by the localization of pleasure in the penis alone, while most women know overall pleasure without doing any apprenticeship at all."

"But during the initiation of a woman, aren't there any physical practices?"

Devi looked at me, amused.

"There are, and it won't be long before you'll discover them. We develop the internal muscles linked to our genitals, the abdominal muscles, and the muscles necessary for the postures. My vagina is as strong as my hand. It knows how to take, to grip, to hold, to open, and to close without the least spasm. It knows how to give itself pleasure through deep contractions. It knows how to become soft as an infant relaxing its muscles. It knows how to make use of the river water and play with the little stones. It knows how to close at the moment of death and open at the moment of life."

16

Devi asked me to go find an armload of small branches and make them into a pile, then to make another pile of medium-size branches, and then a third of large branches. When evening came, on the esplanade, she told me to light the first pile.

The flame grew high in the darkness. The wood crackled, and the fragile, orange embers collapsed at the center of the fire, hollowing out a chimney. We watched this intense burning with wonder, and as soon as the flames diminished, I wanted to feed the fire with some of the thicker branches. Devi stopped me and said to look at the fire carefully. Very soon, the consumed brushwood left only a pile of fragile ash.

"You see, this magnificent short-lived blaze is an image of a sexual relationship between a man and a woman at its best. It's beautiful, intense, and short. A great fire, but there's no avoiding the final embers. Put some branches on the embers."

A few minutes later, a second blaze lit up the sky, but this time, Devi and I carefully fed the fire so that it remained constant. We took great pleasure in feeding it branch by branch. Until dawn, the flame stayed alive, steady and even, and there wasn't a second when our attention lapsed. Then we took our positions and entered into *samadi* until morning. Devi gently rubbed her face and limbs.

"This magnificent fire, which has illuminated our heart all night is the Tantric Great Union of Shiva and Shakti, of Bhairavi and Bhairavi. Adepts identify themselves with the gods and settle in for the duration, which unfolds into mystical ecstasy. Thus, it is important to feed the passionate momentum needed to carry us toward each other with our power and our capacity for wonder. Everything invented by men, women, animals, and plants in the way of amorous play is the branches we will throw into the hearth. But there we will also throw our thoughts, our ideas, our crude desire, and our three impurities.

"The first of these impurities is that which makes us identify pleasure and pain with our limited egos. All sensation is thus reduced to the dimensions of the ego, which makes pain more vivid and pleasure more subdued. The tantrika is free of this association and lets sensation flow in the divine within him.

"The second impurity springs up at the center of consciousness in the form of duality. It engenders fantasies of possession of beings and things. Beginning from the moment when we want some exterior thing, when we want to put our seal on it and call it 'ours,' we lose communication with this being or this thing, and we leave it to rot in the fortress of our possessions. One day, we think of this thing, of this being we've imprisoned by our desire. We go to search for it among the innumerable objects that we have piled up. And we discover to our astonishment that this being or thing is no longer alive, that it must be thrown out. Possession and rejection are one and the same gesture of ignorance.

"The third impurity is as subtle as a very light gauze that flies in the wind. Sometimes it unveils our consciousness, and we have the impression that we are opened enough to ground ourselves in Shiva. Sometimes this gauze casts a light shadow, and our consciousness then suffers by not getting absolute light. It's this subtle impurity that makes our meditation oscillate between unity and duality. Sometimes we grasp our absolute Self. Sometimes we lose it. We are not filled by the divine, and our thirsty consciousness feels deprived. Shiva has only one foot in our pained heart, and sometimes we lose him altogether. Then we feel an exposed emptiness like a freshly opened wound, and even the divine becomes a cause for suffering. That's then we sometimes form obsessive attachments to our spiritual masters. If the latter aren't accomplished, they feed on this, and we become dependent. Our spiritual progress is blocked, our vitality and equilibrium becoming precarious and subject to the whims of the master. This pernicious relationship frequently develops. As soon as simple, deep, and unstrained devotion is transformed into a frenetic relationship, there are attempts by the disciple to manipulate the master, or vice versa, or both at the same time. Through this process, spiritual energy is reversed, and love becomes power.

"Healthy relationships between master and disciple are free of artifice and protocol. Even in ritual, when the master releases his power, the relationship must remain simple. Together they must navigate these accelerations and shifts in power for the relationship to remain fair and true.

"The human hears the human, the human responds to the human, the human is grounded in the human. The divine hears the divine, the divine responds to the divine, the divine is grounded in the divine. When communication goes from one plane to the other, from the human to the divine, there is confusion and impurity, and the communication isn't true.

"In the Great Union ritual, Shakti is adored by Shiva. Their passion traverses all states, all the thirty-six *tattvas*. That is to say, it goes from the earthly tantrika tasting the goddess to divine absorption in Shiva. All these stages are lived in the most intense and complete manner. All human passions and desires must be satisfied during the energetic ascent toward union. No area of desire must be pushed aside, because frustration is contrary to the divine. It is essential that you fully understand each aspect of the ritual so that it can unfold like lightning and not be held up by any confusion. Also, ask me questions if you want to."

"How does the ritual unfold?"

"After sleeping together naked, you on my left, then on my right, then embracing, for three periods of equal length, we take a ritual bath and return to the forest.

"Then you draw on the ground a yantra, a symbolic geometric figure, which will protect the ritual place from all harmful influences, and there you unroll the blanket on which you will throw flowers to make a rug.

"You assemble the offerings of flowers, perfumes, food, and palm wine that we will share over the course of the sacrificial meal. Then you perfume my body and you touch it, beginning at the heart, in the twenty-one places I've shown you. This palpable adoration of the goddess awakens her senses and insures that every organ participates in the great libation. I then enter into the deep continuous sound that, by spreading waves through your body, will awaken all your centers.

"When the vibrations and trembling in you and me come into accord like two musical instruments, we will begin to discover our bodies with the passion of two young newlyweds. In full consciousness, like a child who has never seen a woman, you will look at my face, my breasts, my arms, my hands, my stomach, my genitals, my legs, my ankles, my feet, and, in the same way, you will take in the other side of my body. When my entire image is present in you and you have completely accepted me as the goddess herself, I will take my turn at recognizing you as Shiva.

"Then, we will chant the mantra AUM together. Born in the heart with the A, it rises toward the throat with the U and dies against the roof of the mouth with the M, while its resonance crosses through the fontanel and merges with the sky. When the mantra has united our sonorous essence, we will unite our breathing in the long and deep rhythm that is the measure of Being. With this breathing, we agree to abandon ourselves totally to each other, free of all ordinary sentimental impulses, in a sacred encounter where the three jewels are mastered: the breath, the mind, and the orgasmic nectars. Then alone is there true divine union.

"Then we will be Shiva and Shakti, in the center of the magic yantra. I will enter into your voice, you will enter into mine, and we will recognize each other as divine under the gaze of my master and his Shakti, whose presence and power I will invoke as you do the same. Thus, the power of the two lines will be within us.

"Next, you will offer flowers and sandalwood paste to my *yoni*. Then I will make the same offering to your *linga*. When you are erect as the *linga* of Shiva, and my *yoni* is trembling and parted with desire, we will begin to give ourselves over to the divine play of love. Then, saying the mantra '*Aham*,' 'I am Shiva,' you will honor the goddess with your caresses, your kisses, your tongue, your fingers, your teeth, your fingernails, and the touch of all your skin on mine. Slowly, divinely, you will bring me to the height of desire, and I will do the same for you.

"We will be careful to always stay on the same vibratory plane, each bringing the other up to the level we ourselves have reached. This slow ascent, which includes at least four stages of pleasure, will lead us to penetration, which should provoke immediate orgasm if the rise of excitation occurs in complete harmony and with sufficient power. All the fires of passion, all the erotic games of the animals and plants to whom we must appeal for inspiration and protection, should carry us to a state of extreme intensity. The Great Union is a ritual of power subjected to an extremely vital dynamism, which must not be confused with less charged states.

"Even the *samadhi* of the Great Union retains this scent of divine power. It is as different from the quiescent state as an impassioned lover is from a tranquil one. The greatness of Tantrism is knowing how to use this passionate state to free oneself from the suffering that is at the heart of profane activity.

"Then, as we change position according to our desires,

the night will collect our pleasure and our cries, our whispers and the music of spontaneous love, which knows no hint of possession. Using your mastery of the breath, the mental elements, the sperm, you will offer any number of orgasms to the goddess. Through the control of my internal muscles, my sweet smell, my vital power, my trembling force, I will make you come the same number of times, without ejaculating, each orgasm stronger than the last.

"When at last the divine is totally satisfied with our passion, we will enter into the ultimate phase of the Union. Adopting a stable and unchanging position, seated in a lotus, all of your being deeply rooted in mine, we will enter into *samadhi*. The nature of our pleasure will change, and in the same continuous trembling, my *yoni* closing with all its strength around your *linga*, we will know the final ecstasy. In the lightening rise of the kundalini, we will emit divine nectar, which is entirely different in nature from sperm or the arousal fluids of the woman. This deep emission is the juice of ecstasy. It opens the door of the Infinite to the tantrika, the door of Absolute consciousness, of Being, of the Great Void, which is one of the names of Shiva.

"This step will be the third initiation, which corresponds to the deep passage through the true nature of Self. This passage will inseminate the very depths of your consciousness like seeds dark and speckled with colors as vivid as a poppy's, which will remain at the heart of your medulla. All subsequent practice will bear fruit because of the presence of these seeds. The simple fact of staying in contact with reality, of touching life deeply, will one day provoke awakening, and a field of flowers will blossom in the deepest part of you.

"There is nothing more to do after that but to let things be. To open, to relax, to let the mind rest, to accumulate nothing more, to search no more, to free oneself from doubt and waiting, that thick barrier that keeps the rain and the sun from germinating the deep seeds I will have planted in you."

17

The twelve days that followed were the most peaceful time I spent with Devi. Everything unfolded in presence, leisure, freedom, laughter, and nocturnal dancing. We spent much time playing at the waterfall, as carefree as two adolescents. Strangest for me was the sensation of living so deeply in each other's presence even during the most insignificant activities. This presence, this intense communication, was totally free of mental constraints, plans, or emotional manipulation, as if everything had come together to flow harmoniously within reality.

I experienced a new kind of bond between male and female, between master and disciple. Nothing in the human sphere of sensations was excluded from our relationship, and at the same time nothing consigned to us by habit or routine entered into it. We wasted not a minute on confrontation, dullness, or desire. Nevertheless, the power in play went well beyond that which energizes the most extreme situations of tension or conflict. I had the impression that it was all there, that every human impulse was present, but that all these states played their part within an absolute freedom, remaining latent and unevoked. In this way, their vital force came to nourish each of our acts. There were no outbreaks of anger, desire, passion, sexuality, love, presence, or compassion. Nor was there the resorption of these forces following the short crises we're so accustomed to.

Devi didn't pass from one to the other. There was neither rising nor falling, neither exhaustion nor recharging of energy. These feelings existed simultaneously in her. Her smallest gesture drew upon the entire human palette. It was as if her look were saturated with an ageless humanity, lacking nothing.

The feeling of very deep veneration that I had for Devi freed me in some way from all exterior signs of respect; at the same time, each of my gestures was imbued with it. I had before me at all times a being who seemed to live on all planes simultaneously, and whose spontaneity was such that the earth and sky seemed grateful to her. Her gentleness, power, freshness, wisdom, almost childlike enthusiasm for the world, and supreme knowledge were always obvious and were expressed in the smallest gesture, the least facial expression.

For the first time we slept naked together. Four days on the left, four days on the right, four days embracing. There was no sexual contact between us, but very tender, very full touch, which couldn't be considered asexual either. On the contrary, hour by hour, our bodies seemed to be charged with cosmic electricity so that even brushing lightly against each other made us tremble from head to foot.

During these wonderful days, I experienced the life of the yogi, which wasn't anything like our austere stereotype of it. Still, at the same time, this joy, this freedom, this spontaneity found its source precisely in austerity, solitude, and the fiercest determination. Our levity and freedom from care, our grace and perfect integration into space were a kind of manifestation of the divine running through us. I felt it as a rosy perfume scenting our open consciousness.

These peaceful days were also days of dialogue, which I took advantage of by asking all the questions close to my heart. During the whole first part of my *sadhana*, I had been obsessed by the body of that man found drowned in the river. All sorts of crazy ideas had gone through my head, ranging from the ritual murder formerly practiced by certain Tantric sects to an accident taking place during one of the tests, like the one on the cliff. I had also thought of a panicked flight in the depths of the night, knowing how terrifying Devi could be. I asked her the question directly:

"Are there still human sacrifices in some Tantric rites?"

"Human sacrifice is constant. Men sacrifice themselves by not realizing their absolute nature."

"And ritual murders?"

"I've never seen any. Those are ancient practices."

"What about the death of the man they found in the river?"

"I don't know. I've never heard about it."

"They told me this story in the village, and I imagined that he fell off the edge of the cliff during a test."

"The test of the cliff corresponded to a fear that you had to vanquish. Everyone is different; each test is different. There's nothing systematic in the *sadhana*. Everything happens according to the goodwill of the master, who senses what the disciple needs to come through his fear. Once, I had a disciple whose greatest fear was learning how to read and write. This isn't a subject of fear for us, but for him it represented much more than passing a night with lepers or three nights alone in the heart of the forest. This was a very courageous young man. He would climb down into a pit full of snakes or tigers, but the printed word made him tremble."

"At the beginning, when I spoke to you about the *Vijnanabhairava Tantra,* you told me that the Chinese yogi who had given it to me was an impostor, and I have never really understood why you brought this accusation against this man, who was the first to welcome me along the Tantric way."

"It is difficult to teach. It is difficult to accept or refuse a disciple. The first interview is rarely a contest to see who can be more polite. When you smile, the world seems marvelous; when you attack, a person's true face shows through. That's what's called subtle means, or *upaya.* The special trait of a master is finding what will suffice. You took great intellectual pride in possessing this Tantra. You felt you were part of a rare elite. So that's the spot where I chose to touch you. I don't doubt that this yogi is respectable, and if he passed this essential text on to you, it was, without a doubt, to sow the seeds that are now in the process of sprouting in you. If he hadn't done that, you probably wouldn't be here. If Kalou Rinpoche hadn't accepted you as a disciple and hadn't taught you to practice, you probably wouldn't be here. Everything fits together. Everything is connected and corresponds. The first thing one senses in facing a potential disciple is not his past apprenticeships, his knowledge, his experience, his familiarity with a mental realm, but rather his energy, its ramifications in space, his ability to take curves of great amplitude without being shattered or lost.

"Accumulated knowledge is not important. What matters is to grasp what someone is ready to give up in order to receive the teaching. All teaching is colored as a function of that. To those who lack any base, one teaches the sacred texts. As for those absorbed in the mental, one gives them hardly a sign. They are forced to live the teaching with their whole bodies. I cut off your head. For others, perhaps I would have cut off a leg, or the penis. We all have one part of our body that we wouldn't lose for anything in the world. It's the same for the ritual, for the initiations, the mantras, the meditation supports, the *maithuna*.

"Tantrism remains vital because it has never been systematized. Everything is possible. For some, there is only a single initiation during which everything is transmitted. For others, there are three of them, or five. Everything is suspended, open, unfathomable, and free. Sometimes the goddess is honored by retention and mounting waves of successive orgasms. Sometimes the goddess is honored by the free flow of essential fluids. Sometimes the goddess is honored by a single look. Sometimes the goddess remains invisible and unites with the tantrika only in the absolute solitude of the heart. Sometimes the tantrika carries the goddess within him and has no need at all for an exterior Shakti to accomplish the Great Union rite. It's important to understand that the initiation I am giving you into the Great

Union could be accomplished just as well symbolically, without any carnal contact at all. Its value would be the same. The whole Tantric itinerary can be completed in absolute chastity. Each master has complete freedom to decide. It's also one of Tantrism's great strengths that nothing which makes up being human is rejected. There are no rules, no methods, no way, no effort, no accomplishments, no fruit. Everything happens as if one is letting his own sky be cleared of haze and clouds. The sun, moon, and stars are always there."

"Can you tell me how to practice yoga?"

"The Great Yoga—that is to drink, to eat, to touch, to see, to walk, to sleep, to urinate, to defecate, to listen, to remain silent, to speak, to dream, to love, to sit, to cross the street, to get on a bus, to travel through town and country, sights and sounds, beauty and ugliness without ever being separated from the divine, which is in the self. No type of yoga is better than that which isn't afraid of immersion in reality. Outside of reality, there is not a single trace of the absolute.

"The Great Yoga is like the English grammar that I taught at school. It is very simple. There is a sentence, some words, a punctuation mark. The Great Yoga is very acute perception of the punctuation. We are used to paying attention to the words, but the door to the divine is found in the punctuation. The commas, the periods indicate the pose taken between two parts, between two propositions, between two sentences. The comma, the period—that's infinity. That's the void."

"How do you apply this grammar of yoga to the life of the tantrika?"

150

"Between two breaths, there is a comma. Between two feelings or two ideas, there is a comma. Between one gesture and another, there is a comma. The magic of the Great Yoga is that all life experiences are followed by a comma, and the yogi can continually operate in and drink from the infinite by being conscious of this punctuation. Our life is too often like a text without punctuation. We believe that the words run together to infinity. When we begin to meditate, we are frightened by the huge lava flow of words that pushes us continually forward or to the side of our lives. We feel ourselves bombarded by our chaotic mental activity, which swallows up our punctuation and leaves us exhausted, no longer making sense.

"Bit by bit, the air penetrates our meditation. The magma of words becomes more like a strip of clay that you can stretch between your two hands. All of a sudden, there is a rupture, a silence, a void, a comma, and true life begins. This break allows us to be present, to catch our breath, to enter into the next group of words fully conscious. These moments of emptiness are like rest stops on a long climb. They allow us to realize what we're in the process of doing and to taste it fully. That's yoga. Ascetic exercises in a hidden cave are yoga only if the ascetic can descend to beg for his grain in the town and cross through it in full consciousness. Otherwise, they are only vain austerities. Anyone who can't immerse the entire body and consciousness in life without being thrown off by it is on a sterile path. Continuity is everything in Tantrism. Continual ecstasy, continual divinity, continual life.

"There comes a day in the practice of yoga when the entire reality of the world, all its forces, all its antagonisms begin to run together and to have a single taste and smell. The absolute smells wonderfully good, and its most fetid components are part of this divine perfume.

"Practicing this way is practicing without interruption but with extreme care for punctuation. Practicing intermittently, returning to the ashram after work, is a way of refusing the continuity of mystical experience. The continuity can never be experienced that way, since only a part of the Self returns. Nothing can be divided. There can't be a box for the pleasures of the mind, a box for the pleasures of the body, a box for the divine, a box for violence, a box for those without social standing, a box for the privileged.

"The real way life works is that everything communicates and everything transmits a charge. Fragmentation leads to explosions on the individual and social levels. Everything separate is destined to die out. To be alive is an act of ultimate courage, since to live is to realize how immaterial these divisions and boxes are, and to throw oneself into the great maelstrom. Contrary to what most people think, there is no risk in throwing oneself into the maelstrom, but one can know that only after having jumped. And that's the difficult part, to jump.

"To jump! That's the Great Yoga!"

18

We spent two or three hours a day repeating the mantra AUM in one voice, slow and deep, feeling each low-frequency vibration throughout the rest of the body, like the sound box of a stringed instrument. At first, Devi accompanied us with a gesture signifying the opening of the A in the heart. Her joined fingers opened like a lotus. The sound emerged, grew, and gave birth to the U in the throat, which then blossomed into the resonance of the M in space. Devi had me observe the birds singing in the forest. She relaxed my throat with her fingers, delicately massaging my trachea.

"If you don't understand how the birds sing, the way in which the song makes them shudder and intoxicates them, you can't give life to the mantra. It's necessary to be entirely absorbed in the pleasure of the sound and let it rise naturally until the M becomes energy turning in the mouth, and the spirit of the sound climbs in its fullness to the *bindu* at the top of the skull. From this point on, the sound is no longer silence. It becomes radiance, spreading around you like a robe of pure light. Then it disperses into space and comes to germinate again in your heart. All energy is cyclical. Nothing is lost, nothing disappears, nothing is created. The mystical life is a spiral, a child's pinwheel upon which Shiva never stops blowing. You breathe; Shiva blows. You stop breathing; Shiva sleeps."

We were in the last of the preliminary days. We slept intertwined, and Devi introduced me to a new mystery. Wrapped around each other like two vines before slipping into sleep late at night, we began with a long period of deep breathing, belly to belly. This breathing left me highly intoxicated. Devi had explained nothing to me. At the first embrace, she began to breathe very slowly and I had the impression that she was enclosing me in her belly, that I was becoming a fetus again, and that I was breathing with her. Despite my well-developed rib cage, I still had some sort of reserve that kept me from following her to the end, but little by little, in letting myself go, I underwent this extraordinary experience. To encourage me, or to make my last tensions disappear, Devi slowly caressed my face, throat, ears, forehead, the nape of my neck, and my skull. Her hands, like the rest of her body, let off a heat so intense I felt as if I were melting each time I exhaled. Then she spoke to me in a very soft deep voice while she slid me between her legs:

"The body of Shakti is a garden where the adept, going from one flower to another, breathes the perfume that purifies the heart, making him ardent but free of desire, subtle, but charged with the power of the woman, delicate as a young virgin, but powerful as a snow leopard. In breathing the perfume of the *yoni*, you are intoxicated and recognize the existence of Devi in yourself. Climbing gently, you breathe the nectar of the navel and recognize in yourself the orifice that nourished your embryonic consciousness. Then, very slowly, you climb up between the breasts, and there, you're intoxicated by the ambrosia of the heart of the yogini, which recalls for you your own heart longing to be totally opened. Then, inhaling the breasts, you recognized the perfume of sleep, which descends upon you.

"During your dreams, you realize, thanks to this persistent perfume, that it is the divine who dreams in you. Thus, you can obtain the power to dream in full consciousness and to be fully present, as a yogi is present in his cave, when the tendencies enfolded in your deepest consciousness open. Thus, in dreams, all traces of unsuccessful actions that cause endless regret and obstruct the consciousness rise to the surface, opening out and losing their paralyzing energy. All this negativity then recognizes a point of divine light in itself, which has always been there. This is not a sublimation, or any kind of transcendence, but simply the recognition of how fundamentally everything is saturated with the divine.

"No act loses us; no violence we're subjected to destroys us; no debasement chases out the divine. No one can give us the divine, and no one can take it from us. And we can have access to it at any time by breathing the intimate perfume of the woman, the perfume of the world."

In the arms of Devi, sleep took on the aspect of intense rest, since the body and the consciousness seemed to remain vital and alert. It is a strange experience, feeling so deeply relaxed and so spiritually alive at the same time.

You open your eyes for a moment, and a wave of infinite gratitude comes over you, and then you're plunged again into this awakened sleep.

Each time my eyes opened, Devi's eyes opened too. In the moon's glimmer, I saw her dark look, enlarged by the closeness of our faces. There was always a sort of fundamental smile in her. Her ash-covered body warmed me incredibly. I felt a vital circulation of energy. By breathing her in, I seemed to experience neural pleasure, orgasms in the eyeballs simultaneous with an intense humming in the skull, which spread to the coccyx and the soles of the feet. It was then that I felt the internal heat of the yogis.

By morning, after these magical nights, I felt very much like an animal, like a young bear coming out of hibernation, full of strength and life. Our play at the waterfall had the festive air of a big parade. This approach of a love that doesn't rely on a single emotional fantasy and that seems capable of expanding endlessly is one of the most powerful shocks in the Tantric *sadhana*. It is love without the restrictions or the extreme tensions of passion, without manipulation, without the anguish of continuity, of possession by or of the other. It is a love that ceases to be taken or given, in order to be overwhelmed by the divine.

One day, as we were drying ourselves in the sun on our large, flat, warm rock, I began to think for the first time of life after Devi—of my return to the Western world, of how I was going to survive the separation. I then had the experience of seeing how, in a matter of seconds, this single thought reduced the ecstatic field on which I was living. I felt as if my whole body and consciousness were shrinking, as if I'd been plunged into the head-shrinking liquid of the

Jivaro Indians. And this time, it wasn't a little pebble that landed in the pot, but a big round one, the size of my shrunken head, that Devi threw into the green water of the basin. At the moment of the loud splash, I immediately regained my space.

"The closer an experience of total opening approaches, the more the bodymind struggles. These moments are all the more difficult to go through because the trip toward the ego happens in a flash. You're suspended in the real space of heavenly pleasure, and suddenly, you leap into a cauldron of tar. The experience is unpleasant, but you must get used to it. It is what awaits you until the day when your heart opens completely.

"The embryo knows this anguish. The completely formed infant knows it most when its mother's contractions begin. Birth is a spiritual test equivalent to the awakening and opening of the heart. It is from this combat, from these memories, that the gods are born. Terrifying or kind, they are only products of our consciousness's great struggle to attain life and absolute love.

"Man is afraid of losing himself in the taste and smell of the female genitals, because if his tension and suffering are too great, the memory of his divine life inside the woman can cause a great shock. A rupture makes the armor protecting him from love's reality explode. A door is opened in his hatred, and his suffering grows. In the same way, a woman who fears the man's penis and can't let herself go, adoring it in complete freedom, refuses her own power and obstructs her own consciousness. She also opens the door to negativity. Sexual relations then become combat between two negative forces. Divine play is perverted, its deep meaning goes unrecognized, and one stops being in constant loving rapport with reality.

"We suffer from our absence from the world. The deep consciousness becomes weighted down with each experience, and the universe becomes sad and gray. Loneliness establishes itself, and the prospect of death becomes so terrifying that we spend our time escaping from ourselves into all sorts of artificial and limited pleasures. When we dress ourselves in ashes, we dress ourselves in the dust of the dead, and by penetrating our hearts, we offer them the freedom of finally recognizing the divine.

"The tantrika refuses limited pleasure. He lets his consciousness go back to the source. He recognizes the male and the female in himself. He opens himself to the world and then grasps that time and space, desire, lack of fulfillment, and limited creativity are bogeymen meant for terrified beings. If beings weren't terrified, there would be no gradual approaches to spirituality. If beings weren't terrified, there would be no tests to submit to. If beings weren't terrified, there would be no gods outside of the Self, no paths leading to them, no illusory progress, no metaphysics, no conceptualization of the divine.

"Shivaism offers unconditional freedom to the people of the Kali Yuga, or dark age. Few are capable of grasping it. It burns like a fierce fire, but it takes only a very small opening in the consciousness for the divine to rush in. The divine is like a guest one makes sleep outside. That's not its natural place. It waits patiently to enter until we really want to open a door or shutter part way. That's why we often use the expression 'coming back' to its own home, or 'returning' to the Self. I was pushing your hand into the fire the moment when you were opening your shutter. A second too soon, and you would still bear the marks of the burn."

On the morning after the twelfth night, we meditated, chanted the mantra, and then went down to the river in silence. Three times Devi let the water run over my head, and then we were on our way toward the heart of the forest for the merging of the Great Union. We took only a jug of water, and I wondered how we were going to carry out the ritual Devi had described to me. Where would we find the perfumed oils, the flowers, the palm wine, the sacrificial dishes, the incense, the cushions, the oil lamp, the canopy of purple silk to hang above the divine lovers?

19

I drew the yantra, following Devi's instructions. She had chosen a mossy spot, slightly sunken and protected. She sat down in a lotus position, and I faced her. Devi looked at me for a long time, and as my eyes found their calm in hers I felt tears well up and run down onto my chest. It was an experience of great fullness to which I completely let myself go.

"Those are the rose petals of our bed," Devi said.

When this beneficial flood stopped, Devi asked me to light the incense on the silver tray. She laughed at my bewilderment.

"Children need only their imaginations to create treasures, palaces, music, and perfume. It's enough to see the silver tray and the incense for the nostrils and the senses to be filled with wonder."

Then I saw the tray. I lit the incense. I smelled its delicate sandalwood odor. Devi asked me to offer her the meat roasted with spices and the palm wine. After having tasted each, she put them carefully into my mouth. I experienced their textures, tastes, and smells perfectly. I had lost all sense of play. We were carrying out the Union, the gods providing our imaginations with a fine materiality that quenched our thirst.

Devi asked me to thread the flowers together to make a garland. I made them slide down the string one after the other while she prepared hers. Then came the offering. Devi entered into the sound, and then, without emerging from this state of deep absorption, she indicated to me that it was time to touch her heart and the secret points before perfuming her limbs. On the silver platter, I opened the flasks, their many essences ravishing me.

When that was done, she took her turn perfuming me. Then she emitted a very deep sound of such low intensity that it seemed to be sustaining itself on its own infinite vibration. Without even knowing when the sound was born in me, I realized at a certain moment that I was emitting the same sound and that it was penetrating us totally.

Devi drew me toward her. I began to travel up and down the terrain of her body like a traveler thirsting for infinite slowness. She did the same, and we found ourselves immediately inscribed in each other's consciousness.

When the mantra AUM gave us access to each other's breath and voice, Devi's master and his Shakti responded to our invitation and came to install themselves on the thick cushions. A musician invited by Devi took his *sarod* out of its case while the *tabla* player tuned his two instruments with the help of a little hammer. The *sarod* player turned the pegs of the instrument, tightening or loosening the strings until they were perfectly in tune.

Then I again offered flowers and sandalwood paste. Devi asked the phallus of Shiva to become erect. Facing me, Shakti bathed in a milky glow that seemed to emanate from her skin. The *sarod* player began the slow *alap* (prelude in which the *tabla* doesn't have a part) of a Bhairavi raga, and, bending over Devi, I kissed her lips.

The caresses, the gentle bites, the passionate scratches, the hungry feasting on each other's genitals, the slow curling of light and supple bodies followed one after the other exactly like notes, until the *alap* came to an end.

When we had been brought to a first orgasm by our lovemaking, I entered Devi at the moment the *tabla* began to play. The second orgasm was nearly immediate, and as the intensity of the *raga* unrolled into the night, we rose with the musicians to repeated and uninterrupted heights in the trance.

When the music gave way to silence in the last simultaneous chord, we had taken the yoga posture, totally interwoven in each other. Thanks to Devi, the serpent of the depth unwound itself in one great shudder, and the kundalini took possession of us.

20

In the days that followed the *maithuna* ritual, I came and went, enjoying divine freedom, my bodymind continuing to tremble. I felt like foliage that reality was filtering through. The deep bond connecting Devi and me extended to the entire world, and I spent day and night in a continual state of rapture. Everything took on a startling depth because everything took place in a single space where the ego was temporarily diluted. This presence of total reality left me filled with wonder and free of all concepts. Each movement attested to a deep harmony with the All.

From the morning bath on, I felt myself to be in a state of uninterrupted gratitude. I wanted to bow deeply to the world, to sing out the wonder of each thing. Reality saturated with the absolute never stopped running through me as I ran through it, and nothing was without resonance. As we climbed out of the water and dried ourselves in the sun and air, Devi said to me:

"You see, ecstasy is the natural human state, and the obstacles we create to ecstasy are part of a dictatorial state our thought makes us live in. Ecstasy is simpler than suffering. It smells good. It is present throughout. It is with us always. There is nothing to do and nothing to look for. It's enough to stay totally open and let things occur without worrying about changing their nature. By our being really present, continuously present, all reality becomes a source of joy and happiness.

"You know that the moment for us to take leave of each other has come, and you won't suffer because the bond that unites us doesn't unite us to each other but simply passes through us to extend to the whole universe. You don't belong to me; I don't belong to you. We belong to the world, to the divine, and at this moment we know that with our whole being. Our bond isn't subject to time or space. I will be everywhere you look. You have planted yourself firmly in the heart of the goddess, in my heart, just as the goddess remains in yours, as I remain in yours. We are a divine waterfall for each other where we can bathe ourselves in light and quench our absolute thirst.

"The universe is a great pot that we never stop shaping with our flesh, our hearts, our thought—with all those little things that we love to separate from one another by artifice. But a good potter sinks his hands into the divine and lets the divine take varied forms. He knows that the earth contains the thirty-six modalities of consciousness, and he doesn't spend his time analyzing them.

"While the man thinks, the tantrika makes a pot. While the man confines his consciousness, the tantrika widens the opening of the pot and lets his consciousness experience the void. Distinguishing between what's inside the pot and what's outside is possible only if you forget that a pot needs an opening, without which there is seclusion, darkness, rot, and decay.

"The tantrika widens his pot. He enjoys letting the universe spill in and penetrate it. When he meditates, he experiences a single space. When he undergoes change, he experiences a single space. When he dreams, he experiences a single space, and when he dies, he experiences nothing other than a single space. So for him, there is no difference between meditating, living, dreaming, and dying. To experience a single space—that's absolute love."

Some time later, we went back up toward Devi's hut to share one last meal. The atmosphere was joyous and light. I felt a bit of a pang at the idea of leaving, but I also knew that Devi would be everywhere and that her grace would never leave me.

Devi told me to ask her all the questions I wanted cleared up, and while we drank some good strong tea, she answered them.

"Will the day come when I'll be continually bathed in this state?"

"When the moment comes, your heart will open. The primordial Shakti will appear to you, and you will be bathed in an unalterable joy. Everything will rejoin simplicity. This joy will be no different from what you know at this moment, but it will be without ups and downs, without variations in intensity, and everything will take part in it. You will feel a more or less violent shock, after which the kundalini will no longer rise like a spaceship taking off but will be more like an abundant and constant spring, which endlessly renews itself by circulating through you. Only then will you have received my complete transmission, my last initiation, and the power to transmit the teaching yourself.

"All teaching must be marked with the seal of the heart, and the seal of the heart is what makes Tantrism penetrate all."

"How will I know that my heart is really opened—that it's not my imagination?"

"It's just as easy as knowing whether you've fallen off the cliff or are still on the edge. When you fall, your concepts will be shattered like a bag of bones. When the fire rises in you, you will have more and more trouble reemerging from ecstasy and reality both. You can't be fooled. In the beginning, the ecstasy will come in waves and will subside as it pleases. You will feel moments of intense communion and others that resemble oblivion. But when even the smallest trace of the infinite is allowed into the consciousness, it can't keep from totally emerging.

"The essential thing is not to chase after ecstasy. It arises naturally if your presence in the world remains relaxed, without goals and constraints—free, opened, and light. There is no special practice to keep up. If you want to meditate, meditate. If you want to take a walk, take a walk. If you want to work, work. If you want to practice the *maithuna*, practice the *maithuna*. If you want to withdraw into the forest, withdraw into the forest.

"It's the continuous experience of freedom that constitutes the tantrika's asceticism, not any constraint on the spirit. When ecstasy comes, take it. When it leaves, don't worry. If you let the divine come and go as it pleases, it becomes familiar. If you force it to stay within you or pursue it, it can become terrifying. Let yourself be. Be your own master. Stop all searching, and you will find yourself in the truth.

"When this awakening, this opening of the heart takes place, don't fix it. Don't make it into a success. Let it be dispersed into space. That's the only place where it can reach maturity, which means opening for an entire life. There is never an ultimate stage to be reached. Everything is in constant flux. To let things be and to let things die when the time comes—that's the whole meaning of life. There's nothing else to do. Everything rises up again from absolute freedom. Nothing fixed, nothing heavy, nothing definitive. No closed image of the divine, no dogma, no belief. Do not be for or against a single one of the ideas the faithful habitually attach themselves to out of terror. Death, *karma*, and reincarnation are only empty words used by those who haven't realized the divine. All concepts, dogmas, beliefs are like the flesh and bones of the dead. With time they end up as part of the earth again. As for the secret teachings, they remain secret simply because those who hear them or read them without having the necessary open mind don't understand them. It's beautiful to see the letters printed on the page. They see and understand only what their minds and hearts can grasp.

"The great Tantric sages have written down their thoughts. Despite that, the Tantric spirit of secrecy has never been broken. It's like a charm that keeps unprepared eyes from discovering territories they would disfigure by their thoughts. The divine opens or closes the eyes, frees or obstructs the ears and the understanding of listeners.

"We speak to help adepts recognize what they already vaguely know. Those who don't know, don't understand the teaching. In any case, know how unimportant the words are. What's perceived directly is the heart."

Devi stood up. She went with me to my hut and watched me collect my things. I offered her my knife, which she liked using so much. She offered me her small red necklace with the tiny bells that chimed wonderfully when we practiced the Great Union.

Devi took me in her arms and, with infinite tenderness, held me close. This embrace lasted a long time. When we looked at each other, I was surprised to see that her eyes, like my own, were filled with tears. She smiled and said in her softest voice:

"Who would we be if we refused emotion?"

"If my mind is filled with doubts, if the opening doesn't take place, can I come back to see you?"

"I have given you gold. Keep this gold within yourself until it melts. Then you will have a dream. Your heart will open completely, and the gold will fall like fine rain in your consciousness. Coming back would serve no purpose. The mountains are vast. Freedom is great. I come, I go."

I put my pack on my back. Devi rested her hand on my head and caressed my face. I kissed her hand and crossed the esplanade. As I was about to take the path that descended to the village, Devi called to me:

"Go by yourself, carry Devi within you, take your interior silence as master, and be free."

I adjusted my pack, made three great bows, and rushed down the path to the village.

With great joy, I found Ram again. He offered me tea and looked proudly at me. When I took my leave and gave him enough money to cover taking provisions and necessary goods up to Devi, Ram smiled, a little uncomfortably, as if he'd been saving a big surprise for me.

"Each week, for more than a year, I've been bringing Devi what she needs. I sit in her hut, we share a meal, we talk, she tells me things, and me, I come back down and serve tea to those who want it and say nothing."

"She's a sorceress who feeds on dead bodies and pushes men off the top of the cliff!" I said, laughing.

"That's right!" exclaimed Ram with an angelic smile. "She's terrifying, with her bloodshot eyes!"

"And the man found dead in the river?"

"There has never been any dead man in the river. I think it is you. Haven't you seen your body floating down it?"

Ram went with me as far as the bus stop, and with a respectful smile I said my goodbyes to this budding tantrika who had fooled me so well.

EPILOGUE

When I returned to Paris, the ecstatic moments lived with Devi left a lingering impression for a few months, which was then replaced by a feeling of loss. I understood why Devi said that a mystical experience had to find its fulfillment in one's return to society. Ordinary life is simultaneously a marvelous master and a constant barometer of spiritual realization. The occasions for feeding one's ego are incessant, the frictions of personality continue, the frustrations and desires are no less. And it's only when one begins to function with a certain interior harmony in relation to this frenzy that the fruit of the teaching reaches maturity. I tried to remember Devi's advice: not to lose myself in a frenetic quest or internal tension. I tried regularly to be fully conscious of the thirty-six *tattvas*. I succeeded in stealing from life a few days of joy and profound peace interspersed with passions of all sorts, which were sometimes useful for the great fire that the tantrika tends day after day, and sometimes consumed me and drew me further away from serenity.

After my book *Nirvana Tao* came out in the United States, I was invited to teach Buddhism, Tantrism, and literature at some American universities. I remained there for eight years. And it was precisely during this period, which I spent so closely involved in the texts, the ideas, and the history, that I lost the most important part of what I had experienced with Devi. Many times I was tempted to return to India and see her again, but I knew that I would never find her.

Following these periods of tension, there were sometimes moments of peace and communication, of powerful energy mounting, often to the limit of tolerability. They were followed by a very dark period.

There was a deep antagonism between the academic approach and the *sadhana*, or the way of realization. Finally, I became aware that, thanks to studying the texts, I was going to die stupid. It was by rereading Lao Tsu's *Tao Te Ching* that I came to the decision to no longer teach:

> The one who devotes himself to learning
> acquires something daily.
> The one who devotes himself to the Tao
> divests of something daily.*

I returned to France and gradually won back my serenity. I abandoned this compulsion that pushed me to always discover new texts, new perspectives. I concentrated on

*Gallimard Editions, 1967.

the present, on being fully conscious of each moment, and bit by bit I again found that simplicity I had known with Devi.

The ecstasies often stopped just short of my boundary, as if I were a pot suddenly filling and in danger of spilling over onto reality. These regular flashes opened me more and more, and I felt that something was preparing itself without knowing exactly what. I sometimes had the feeling that this overflowing would destroy me or lead me to madness—or, quite the opposite, a feeling of great peace and deep connection with reality.

Thanks to Devi, I had felt a harmonious surge of kundalini, but I also knew that many mystics experience wild and sometimes terrible surges of this legendary energy, represented by a serpent and called "The Coiled One." Nevertheless, little by little, my anguish dissipated. The tensions in my consciousness relaxed to the point where I abandoned all searching and stopped waiting for whatever it was—without, for all that, ceasing to practice full consciousness through the *tattvas*.

This renunciation opened an enormously calm and harmonious realm to me. I finally succeeded in letting myself be, as I had let myself be at Devi's side. I began to feel her presence, which sweetened the days and nights. I had the sensation of becoming a sort of funnel into which all reality poured.

On December 23, 1993, I was awakened by a dream that completely changed my life. Kalou Rinpoche and Devi appeared to me. Kalou Rinpoche held me close. I felt an intense warmth. Devi, standing a few meters away, wore that magnificent, radiant smile of hers that had always overwhelmed me. My heart opened as if an implosion had taken place and left a gaping hole in my chest. First this void swallowed up the last book I had read, *The Teachings of Ma-tsu,** then all the others, back to the first book given me on my sixteenth birthday, the *Bhagavad-Gita*, which was engulfed and disappeared into my heart. I awoke. At this instant, I felt the kundalini rise. The energy spread out like a sort of internal tidal wave, beginning from the bottom and rising with a shudder into space after having traveled through all the chakras. But the energy also spread like a widening sphere around the Self. I was prey to the same joy, the same plenitude I had felt at the moment of the Great Union with Devi. I knew that I had just received my last initiation.

> When I haven't lived Awakening, I desire it
> When it occurs, fusion takes place
> Experience and experiencer are one
> They are distilled in Absolute Reality

The months passed, and the rain of gold that Devi had spoken of never stopped falling on me. The slow maturation process began. I lived simultaneously in ecstasy and in reality. The Self was opened, rushing out in all directions in space, like an internal big bang, after which, following the great Shivaic cycle of expansion and retraction, it returned to the center of the heart like an infinite breath.

Les Entretiens de Mazu, Ch'an master of the eighth century, introduction, translation and notes by Catherine Despeux, The Two Oceans, Paris, 1986.

A bit later, I decided that the time to transmit what I had received had come. I returned to Los Angeles upon the invitation of a Tantric center, and there, for the first time, I taught. This had nothing in common with my university teaching. I felt Devi's presence strongly, and I saw in the faces of those seated around me that words came not from the intellect but from the heart. Following that experience, I opened the Tantra/Chan meditation center in Paris and began my account of this long initiation.

The opening of the meditation center corresponded to my certainty that the teachings of Shivaic Tantrism, in their simplicity and depths, responded marvelously to the hopes, possibilities, and expectations of women and men today.

We all feel that we must find an antidote to the frenzy in which we live, but for all that we are not ready to adopt beliefs and practices that are culturally foreign to us. In Tantrism, we do not go toward some external thing. On the contrary, we direct ourselves toward our core, our own minds. Tantric practice demands nothing more than this return to the Self. To know, to observe, and to calm ourselves, we don't have to take recourse in any belief whatsoever. Everything is born of the mind and returns there. Shiva and Shakti are born there. We are image and reflection at the same time. By observing the mind we will find there all that we have lost to the exterior: peace, tranquility, the strength to act without being subject to filters or limitations that we have accepted or created, the power to fully communicate with life.

The means for knowing our minds are meditation and the practice of full consciousness. In Tantrism, meditation is very simple. There are no supports, no visualizations, no complicated mantras, no fetishes concerning posture. You sit on a comfortable cushion or on a chair. You calm down. You breathe peacefully, without forcing anything, and you observe. Ideas run by very quickly. You do nothing to slow down this relentless rhythm. You simply take note of the degree to which the mind is racing out of control. For many, it already comes as a huge surprise to see that we can be conscious of this incessant bombardment. Little by little, after three or four meditation sessions, the sitting, the calm, the fact that we are there waiting for nothing, not competing, without a single goal except to be open, to breathe, to feel, brings about in us a strong sense of well-being.

The sessions last an hour at the Tantra/Chan center. We practice the *sarangi* relaxation. We release the energies of the body with a few simple exercises, and then we sit down to hear a talk on Tantrism. Following that, we meditate for half an hour, after which we exchange viewpoints and ask questions. In order for the practice to change our way of living and perceiving the world, it's important to make an effort and compel ourselves to meditate each day. Very quickly, the pleasure and the calm that come over us will make it so we don't need to force ourselves to meditate. That will happen naturally, like being drawn to a source of pleasure. Deep well-being restores communication between our minds and bodies as well as the potential of our active and emotional life and the quality of our relationships with others. This pleasure has the particular advantage of always being available, since it depends only on itself.

While everything else in life is an occasion for measuring oneself against others and putting on performances, meditation opens a space where there is nothing to prove.

We are there simply to know ourselves, to accept ourselves unconditionally, and to love ourselves without making judgments on what we do or think. We communicate with all our energies without dismissing anything. All energy is precious. Anger, jealousy, violence, and negativity are just as acceptable as their counterparts that we consider positive.

By no longer labeling and classifying our impulses, we gain access to a fabulous reserve of energy we can use for meditation and for paying attention to the world. There is no progress, in the sense that we apply that term to a sport or a game. Everything can happen very quickly if we simply agree to sit down in complete freedom. There is nothing to learn, no texts or esoteric principles to study. It's enough to let oneself be free from all mental and physical constraints. The single indispensable thing is to have the desire to know oneself, to take full advantage of life, and to release oneself from suffering.

To meditate in a group, two times a week if possible, makes the beginning of meditation easier. In opening up, one benefits from the energy created by the concentration of the others. It will then be easier to practice alone. Through discussion, one finds the answers to questions that arise naturally and discovers what the others feel deep within themselves. The candor with which we speak is astonishing. It rises instantly with the openness produced by meditation.

From the beginning, meditation practice is accompanied by full consciousness, which makes us discover a marvelous thing: each day, in no matter what life, there are numerous occasions for wonder and for feeling joy and fullness.

It's enough to be attentive. Usually, on the moment of awakening, the mind takes up its furious rhythm before we can enjoy the slightest bit of tranquility. We get up, the mind goes full speed, and life escapes us. We do everything mechanically. While our hands act and our legs carry us, while we prepare our breakfast and wolf it down, sometimes adding in a third activity, we aren't fully conscious. We eat our toast, drink our coffee, think about what we are going to do, listen to the news, leaf through a magazine, jump into the shower, etc.

Anyone can experience full consciousness from the moment of waking onward. Those who try find a surprising pleasure in it. Each activity carried out with attention and calm leaves an impression of fullness, which has an influence over our whole day. To get up and eat breakfast, fully conscious, takes no more time than letting ourselves go on at our usual frenzied pace; exactly the opposite. That doesn't mean that we become deaf and mute, cut off from the life around us, tense and concentrated on our toast. It means that we make full use of all that we are given.

At first we will have a hard time maintaining this consciousness for very long stretches. But if, over the course of the day, we can say to ourselves, "I walk; I breathe; I am here completely; I am aware of the temperature, the nature of the sky, the movements of my body, of a face, the trees, an opening," then all life's experiences will be transformed. We will find occasions everywhere for living fully, for communicating with the environment, with others, and with the Self.

The whole art of Tantric practice is to develop this presence in the world, which meditation deepens daily. You find yourself enjoying things that until then didn't seem the least bit interesting. You note with surprise how this opening completely transforms your quality of life and interactions with others. All of a sudden, you will have created an empty space in yourself, a sort of park where the trees, the flowers, the pools, the shade, and the light will allow you to relax and let others enter.

We are all proud of having acquired, through experience, a strategy for living that determines our relationships with others and allows us to survive. We spend a good part of our time refining this process and testing it. We are constantly reinforcing the ego, trying to get to the end of daily trials. The more we brace ourselves to resist it, the harder the world seems. But when we agree to let go of everything fixed, we discover a peaceful energy that little by little frees us of all strategy. We discover that being open and present allows for everything heard, everything said, everything given, everything received. The tantrika lets be and lets himself be. It's a matter of refusing to be manipulated or to manipulate others. There's no longer confrontation between fragile forces but an open space where things can happen in a surprising way.

However difficult our lives, we daily pass up very deep pleasures that could change our relationship to the world and allow our bodies and thoughts the freedom they need to blossom. No one can control our lives twenty-four hours a day. In the most constricted circumstances, you can find a space where you can get a taste of freedom. As soon as that point of light, however small it may be, establishes itself in our lives, we have begun the process of deep internal transformation, which nothing and no one can hinder.

Practice will change our perspective and our way of achieving happiness. We will need to have much less and to be much more. Gradually, this desire to be will replace the objects of happiness we have created that aren't always attainable. More and more we will notice the infinite number of small things to which no one has special rights and to which we have access at any given moment.

The peace and tranquility provided by the experience of full consciousness will continue to grow, and difficult external circumstances will no longer seem so bad. Much of our tension, stress, and anguish will give way to this wave of lucid attention, which is full consciousness. The inescapable part of negative emotions and situations also depends on our degree of openness. With practice, a growing miracle begins to take root in the everyday. Everything that the mind has tied into knots, it can untie. At our core, there is an empty place—inalienable, pure, and free—to which we can have access if we want it. We will discover the major importance of feminine values, coming from openness, nonviolent communication, and love, which are Tantrism's source, and we will reintegrate them into our everyday lives. We will discover silence, space, and peace. This change begins at the center of the Self and can then extend out toward the exterior. It is the source of profound transformation.

Without this radical transformation in our outlook and daily experience, it is obvious that pursuing initiation into the Tantric sexual practices is futile.

We domesticate the void, learn to enjoy it, and make it an important part of our everyday life. When we no longer fear it, an unlimited and fundamental freedom remains: that of our own minds.

Thanks to the simple, timeless techniques of Tantrism, meditation will no longer be a moment of peace and calm, stolen from a hectic life. We will see that this state is not a digression and that it spills out of the framework of practice to become part of everyday life, even to the point of entering our dreams.

Today, I have the feeling that all contact, all human relationships, all everyday events come to be inscribed in this open space by practice. To live fully, to be totally present in the reality of our world, to write novels, to publish other authors, to taste the thousand pleasures of life are all part of the way. Withdrawing into the Self, spiritual obsession, and being closed to others are signs of a spiritual development that has gone astray and reached an impasse.

To free up what's blocking the mind and body, we also offer Indian massage at the center. Influenced by thousands of years of Tantric culture, it draws upon deep knowledge of the mind and body and their interconnections, energy channels, and vital points. A science, an art, and a kind of therapy all at the same time, it frees the deep, joyous, open, and luminous being that is hidden away in each of us.

With one hand on the chakra of the heart, the masseur relaxes the head and neck. The body is then rubbed with warm essential oils to revitalize the skin and relax the muscles. Then begins a very slow overall massage, starting at the shoulders and in one continuous wave moving to the soles of the feet, then reversing the process. The masseur is at the center of the body. His fingers move along the energy channels, varying their pressure and pausing on the vital points, which they relax, resulting in deep abdominal breathing and release. These peripheral sensations move to the interior of the body, touching each internal organ and setting off a powerful harmonization of energies. With a shudder, this is transferred to the entire body, producing general relief in each cell's pleasure at feeling alive, a relaxed mind, an intense warmth, and a sudden suppleness in the diaphragm and the muscles.

At this stage, the massage becomes a double meditation, total presence in the self and in the joy of feeling alive. It is a return to the peace that has never left us but that we have forgotten.

These practices—the deep work of opening, of confidence, and of exchanges—all release accumulated negative energies and allow us to rediscover harmony, fullness, and the freedom to be, delighting in total communication with the universe and reality.

Each day I pay homage to my wonderful masters, and I try to perpetuate the simplicity and the beauty of their teaching.

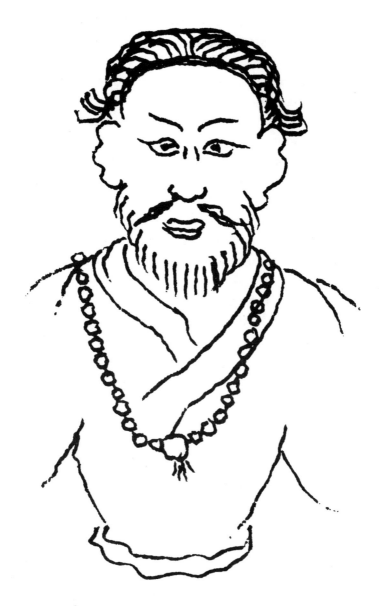

2405

Portrait of Daniel Odier
by Kalou Rinpoché

If you would like to receive information about the Tantra/Chan meditation center activities and retreats, please contact:

Tantra/Chan
15 rue Bénard
75014 Paris
FRANCE
phone: (33) 1 45 42 38 37
fax: (33) 1 45 42 64 46

Jody Gladding is a poet and translator who studied at Cornell and Stanford Universities. Her first book, *Stone Crop,* appeared in the Yale Younger Poets Series. She lives in Vermont.